Stories of the Unborn Soul

ALSO BY ELISABETH HALLETT

In The Newborn Year: Our Changing Awareness After Childbirth
Soul Trek: Meeting Our Children on the Way to Birth

Stories of the Unborn Soul

✦

the mystery and delight of Pre-Birth Communication

Elisabeth Hallett

Writers Club Press
San Jose New York Lincoln Shanghai

Stories of the Unborn Soul
the mystery and delight of Pre-Birth Communication

Writers Club Press
an imprint of iUniverse, Inc.

For information address:
iUniverse, Inc.
5220 S. 16th St., Suite 200
Lincoln, NE 68512
www.iuniverse.com

Acknowledgments of copyrighted material appear on the References page

ISBN: 0-595-22361-3

Printed in the United States of America

Dedicated to all the people who have so generously allowed me to share their stories. By revealing your experiences of pre-birth communication and your memories of the soul world, you make this planet a better home for souls already here and others on the way.

"*Of course, no reasonable man ought to insist that the facts are exactly as I have described them. But that either this or something very like it is a true account of our souls and their future habitations—since we have clear evidence that the soul is immortal—this, I think, is both a reasonable contention and a belief worth risking; for the risk is a noble one. We should use such accounts to inspire ourselves with confidence; and that is why I have already drawn out my tale so long.*"
—from the Phaedo, the last conversation of Socrates

Contents

Editorial Method

A few words about names and notes

Most of the people who shared stories for this book have allowed me to use their real first or full names. Pseudonyms are identified with an asterisk.

Endnote numbers indicate that you will find additional information in the Endnotes at the back of the book.

1

The Shiver Sign

The story began...

> A few months ago, my fiancé and I were lying in bed and simply relaxing. We began kissing and were both inspired to move on to bigger and better activities. All of a sudden, I had the most beautiful, warm, and tingly feeling. I knew that I had felt a child, our child, in the room with us. I immediately stopped Rob and said, "If we make love right now, we are going to have a baby." I was surprised when he replied, "I know." We felt very similar things and at the same time. It was like a wash of a loving, powerful, and familiar presence over us...

As I read Jill's story, a shivery tingle rippled over me. I've come to think of that shiver as a rush of recognition—the soul's "Yes!" response to something that rings true, something that feels electric with meaning. Since I began exploring Pre-Birth Communication almost twenty years ago, I've been privileged to receive hundreds of shiver-inducing stories from people around the world.

What is Pre-Birth Communication? It is the sense of contact with a child yet to be born. The contact may come in a dream, a vision, an inner voice, a hovering presence, or in many other ways. What's central is the feeling that we have touched and been touched by another consciousness, an unborn soul. These experiences are mysterious, joyful, and deeply moving. What they tell us can change the way we see our children and ourselves.

Such contacts are not rare. Though they come most often to mothers or mothers-to-be, they also happen to fathers, grandparents, adoptive parents, other family members, friends, and birth attendants. We seldom hear about them for a simple reason: it's scary to reveal an experience that contradicts the common view of reality. As one woman said, "I have been reluctant to share these experiences, mostly out of fear that people would think I was completely nuts."

All too often, the lack of validation keeps people from telling their stories. And for that very reason, each story shared is doubly precious. Validation is not "proof," but that attitude of respect (from our partners, our friends, the society around us) that says: Your experience, whatever it may ultimately mean, is important and real and worth telling.

One day last summer, I was showing a new friend over our century-old farmhouse. We climbed the stairs to the landing, where I explained, "This is where my father had his study –"and at that moment, simultaneously, the two of us felt a shower of invisible electric rain, the tingles of an unmistakable presence. I realized later that this was a profoundly validating event for me. Like Jill and Rob simultaneously sensing the presence of their unborn child, a shared experience gives us confidence to believe in what we feel. And though such moments may be rare, validation comes in other forms as well.

For many people, just to learn that someone else has had a similar experience is freeing. Kara, whose story is told in Chapter Twenty-One, says: "Thank you so much for giving me the chance to 'come out of the closet' with this! It has been an amazing transformation for me to discover that there are many women and partners who have had these same kinds of experiences and feelings!"

What kind of world is it if these things are true?

It was almost by accident that I stumbled into the study of pre-birth communication. Several years after my first child was born, I was working on a book about postpartum experiences when I noticed an unexpected pattern. Many parents emphasized that their connection with their baby had begun long before the birth. They told of sensing contact and communication during pregnancy, and even before conception.

I was hooked! I had to learn more about this possibility, and my interest was heightened by the fact that I was hoping to have a second child in spite of fertility problems and miscarriages. Exploring the mystery of pre-birth communication led to writing and publishing *Soul Trek: Meeting Our Children on the Way to Birth*. This book and others,[1] along with the information-spreading power of the internet, brought increased awareness—and many more reports of pre-birth communication. It is a delight to share a new collection of these compelling stories.

Each story is like a piece of colored glass, a kind of magic lens. Looking through it, you may see a world very different from the world you are used to, the one you've been told is real. Some stories challenge the boundaries of what we imagine is possible—and I think it is healthy to have these mental boundaries stretched now and then.

Although many experiences are related in terms of a specific faith, I do not place a religious frame around the collection as a whole. Connecting with your unborn child can be a powerful spiritual experience, but it is also natural and within everyone's reach. It is as normal as connecting with those who have walked through life's other door.

The story that happens to *you* is the one that changes your world. But there is a gentle power in these accounts of what others have experienced. I remember the exact moment when I became aware of how they have affected me. I was crossing the laundromat parking lot, sunshine warm on my back, carrying a load of laundry toward the car, when the most unlikely sensation filled me…There's a kind of cake you bake, poke holes in it while it's warm and pour in the sweet syrup. Now, I'm naturally a questioner and skeptical to the core, but I suddenly felt just like one of those cakes, saturated with the significance of all these stories. Though I know that illusion and wishful thinking are a portion of our experience, still the evidence of soul's existence before conception and after death seems to me undeniable.

So I invite you to explore this view of life with me, through stories that provide not proof but possibilities to stir our imagination. Imagine that these things are true:

We are souls that exist before we are conceived.
Before conception, we can communicate with our future parents.
We participate in coming to an agreement;
our decisions are mutual and can be changed.
We can announce our arrival
and make our presence known during pregnancy,
even interact in ways that let our parents get to know us before we are born.
As children, we may remember our pre-birth life
and be aware of siblings yet to come.
Family links are enduring; ancestors take an interest in new births
and may act as guides and guardians of the arriving soul.
We can see echoes of other lives together,
and perhaps plan the next act in the long-running play of our existence.

Stories of pre-birth communication give us tantalizing glimpses of our soul's pre-existence. But another window is beginning to open on the unknown land before this life. There are people who remember it, and they are courageously sharing memories long held secret.

2

Soul Memory

"I am curious if there are many people who actually remember their experiences before birth. I have felt very alone for many years, but have considered myself blessed just the same."

—*Monica*

There is an invisible tribe in the world—a tribe of people who have grown up with memories of pre-existence. Whether they describe it as a place, a time, or a state of being, they locate it not just before birth, but before identifying with a physical body. They remember existing as soul.

These people have begun to discover each other and to realize they are not alone. They are sharing stories that in many cases have been kept secret for decades. It is moving to listen in as they describe the loneliness they've experienced, and their relief at finding others like themselves.

"It was confusing growing up with this experience and not knowing what it meant," says Australian Michael Maguire. As a child, Joelle was met with disbelief when she described memories that she assumed were shared by everybody. Wistfully she notes, "I never said anything again for fear of being laughed at." It was fifty years before she spoke again of her memories.

On the surface, soul memory stories are surprisingly individual, but there are deeper similarities among them. Most people begin their account with a disclaimer: language cannot fully express what they remember. They often use the word "indescribable," while telling of an existence filled with peace and a profound sense of connection with all that is. Some recall the presence of a bright, loving being. Some remember looking upon the planet as if from a vantage point in space, and many speak of their reluctance to take up earth life. When describing others present with them, they often mention that communication was telepathic.

While some remember choosing elements of their life, many do not. Some have memories of being in the womb, while others feel as though they passed in a flash from the soul world to wake in their baby form. Michael Maguire compares it to waking from anesthesia:

> I can clearly remember being in the spiritual, and then suddenly finding myself on Earth trapped in a baby's body. It's a bit like having an operation. One moment you're in an operating theatre counting back from ten; the next you find yourself in the recovery room. The major difference is that when you have an operation, you're drowsy before and after the operation. With my experience, I was fully mentally alert before and after the transition to Earth.

Throughout this book, soul memories shed light on the mystery of our origin. The five stories in this chapter transport us to an altered state, a very different existence—but is it really unfamiliar? Or does it resonate to something we too have known?

Joelle: A Place Indescribable

> I seem to remember many things from my birth and before, but as I am getting older they are fading. I find a real need to pass it on. I'll start with the earliest feelings I had. When I got sleepy or rested or was ill, I felt like there was a film around me. I could see it, and I

felt enclosed but not scared. I would reach to touch it but couldn't quite reach.

That feeling was one of my first memories. After I went to nursing school, I realized that maybe what I was seeing was when I was in utero, and for a long time I thought everyone remembered being in the womb. The feeling of being enclosed faded when I was in my thirties.

In my thirties, my aunt told me a story of my birth that my mother had never revealed to me. It was a home birth; Mom waited too long and there was a snowstorm and they couldn't get out. She had a long, difficult labor and I was breech. When I finally came out I was almost black and not breathing. My aunt, thinking I was dead, wrapped me in a towel and put me in another room. Finally a midwife arrived. They told her I was dead, but she looked at me and gave me a shot and did a few things and then I started to cry.

I remember before, being in a place indescribable. It's peaceful there, quiet, other people are with me. They are one. We are one. Not male, not female—I can see it in my mind's eye but I can't describe it. There are no voices but I hear words. Someone says, "There's a body, the person who had it felt it was too difficult a life and changed their mind." If I want it I have to go now, now. I hesitate, I hear a voice near me say, "No, it's too soon, too soon, wait a while," but I can't wait, I must go back. Someone says, "Decide now."

Next thing I know I'm in a crib, looking at a wall. I'm about six months old. I see a face, I hear a voice but I don't understand it. But it has a nice smile.

I had these memories of being in a quiet place since I was little. Now I can picture them in my mind's eye when I meditate, or in dreams. As a young child I thought they were a real place, and I didn't know what it meant. I would tell my family, but after a few times they looked at me strangely, like, "What planet are you from?" So I never said anything again for fear of being laughed at. As I got older I tried to put the memories out of my mind. I feel these things are to be told. People need to know, and I think that is why I remember so much—so I can comfort people and give hope, because there is nothing to fear.

Michael Maguire[1]: I will be returning home

I remember standing in a dark space. There was another person standing to my right, and like me, he was waiting to be born into the physical world. There was an older person with us who could possibly be a guide, since he answered my questions and stayed with us until we left.

There were no emotions associated with the prospect of being born. There were no sensations either, such as hot or cold. I felt completely content with myself and my environment. The darkness I was in was not like being in a darkened room; it had depth and perspective, and I could clearly see everything around me. It was kind of like standing in outer space and viewing the earth from a distance. However, I sensed that we were standing on some sort of plain.

Behind us was a crowd of people, but they weren't clear to our vision like the two people standing next to me. In front of us and approximately thirty degrees below us, we could see the earth with the facial images of two couples.

I spoke to the other person next to me briefly, but I can't remember what was said. I remember talking to the older man. When we communicated, it wasn't with spoken words but with a form of telepathy. We communicated with thought transfer but we heard the words clearly as if they were spoken.

I asked the older man who the people were behind us and he replied that they were waiting to be born but they weren't ready yet. I asked him what was that in front of us and he replied that what we were looking at was Earth. I then asked him who those people were whose images appeared on the earth and he replied that they were going to be our parents. I didn't know which parents we were each going to end up with. The older man conveyed to us that it was time to go. The other person standing next to me walked forward and disappeared from my sight. I was told that it was my turn and I walked forward.

Suddenly I found myself lying in a hospital nursery with other babies around me. I still had my normal thought processes at this stage. I noticed three people standing at the foot of my bed, and I immediately recognized two of them as my parents. They looked exactly as their image appeared on the earth. The other person was my older brother, but I didn't know this at the time. I remember lying on my back looking around and thinking this must be Earth. I tried to stand up and found I couldn't, since I was now trapped in a baby's body.

My father, who knew nothing of my experience, often talked about the first time they came to the hospital to see me. He said I stared so hard at the three of them that he thought my eyes were going to pop out.

I was born in 1965 and man wasn't able to view the earth as I saw it, until astronauts went to the moon. As a child, when I first saw the photos of the earth taken from space, it was exactly as I remembered it. I can also remember that, while still in the spiritual, the physical world seemed as unreal as the spiritual does from the physical perspective.

Kathy, another person with soul memories whom we will meet in a later chapter, had a parallel experience: "My mother made such a big deal of the first men walking on the moon and told me to watch and exclaimed, 'Oh, that's what the earth looks like from outer space!' I thought she was off her rocker. Hadn't she seen what the earth looked like from outer space before? Ah well, that was before I realized I was the weird one!" Michael continues his account:

Up until I was about thirteen, I could remember everything that was spoken, word for word. As a child I freely told other children what happened, because I thought it was natural for someone to have such an experience. I only learned of its uniqueness when I could find no one else who had a similar experience and after continually having my memories discounted by others as imagination.

I have no memories of life in the womb. I can remember clearly being in the spiritual, and then suddenly finding myself on Earth trapped in a baby's body. I can't recall anything before being in the dark space; it's as if I suddenly was. The only memories that have faded for me concern precisely what words were said and the order of the conversation. I think I joined my physical body when I found myself in the hospital nursery. I didn't have a choice of when

I was going to enter my body or which pair of parents I was going to end up with. If I was granted a choice, it would have been before anything I can remember.

I feel that I'm only on a journey here, and when I die, I simply will be returning home. I feel that the spiritual world is my real home.

Marilyn: Looking eagerly upon Earth

I've always had an intense propensity to the supernatural, especially prophetic dreams and utterances, which my parents tried hard to beat out of me as a child. My mother often laughed at my "imagination" when I would dare tell her, as a preschooler, of my journey here.

I have memories of pre-conception, choosing the time-line I wanted to be born into and choosing my parents. I know why I came (the earth phase is where spirits become souls) and what I am to become through this life. I also have an inkling of what I am to become in the next life. I actually remember being in God's presence, intense light filled with love. Other spirits, like myself, were being created all around me as living, breathing, thinking, speaking flashes of light matter, directly out of the heart of God.

I was looking eagerly upon Earth as a blue ball on a black background, seeing, and at the same time knowing a journey through it was an honor of the highest caliber to my father, God. As I beheld it, I knew it is the testing ground of all testing grounds for all eternity. It distinguishes forever who is worthy to be leaders in the ever-expanding sphere of God's universes with all its civilizations and cultures.

I remember seeing Earth's time zones, from pre-history to its termination, grid across its sphere like time zones in a phone book. There I was, choosing my life, its time zone, my destiny and my parents.

The journey here was like a flash, and I remember some of my experiences in the womb. My mother confirmed them before she passed away. I remember learning to speak as clearly as I thought, and asking my mother if I wasn't adopted because I was physically nothing like anyone in my family!

Ross Willingham: Such love, joy, and happiness

I have carried a pre-birth memory for as long as I can remember. The following account sounds as though it were full of biblical clichés, but there are no other words to express this experience. Here is my feeble attempt:

I remember a "room" that seemed to be a basement of some type. Steps led from above down into this room, which had no ceiling, no floor and only one wall. The wall was made of rock and the steps were a sandy white color. The room held what I remember to be myself and countless others packed together very tightly—yet even so, we were without form and had no beginning. We had been in that room from what seemed like the beginning of time—but this also seemed like only a few moments.

Periodically, a "being," also without specific features, would "walk" down the stairs. The room was full of incredible excitement and joy at the appearance of this being. Everyone in the room had the desire to be "chosen" and to go along with this being. Each time, the being would select one of "us" (and only one) and "it" would carry us up the stairs. There is simply no way to describe this being.

However, there is much to tell about the duration of the stay in that room. This is where more biblical clichés come along. All of us were devoid of any shape or form that could be identified or described. I had no eyes, yet I could see. I had no ears, yet I could hear. Time stood still, yet time passed quickly.

There was such amazing anticipation of going with this individual that it seemed like an eternity, yet in other ways it seemed to be only a few minutes. The anticipation was filled with joy at the appearance of the being and yet such disappointment that only one was chosen each time. I remember the occasion I was "selected" and was carried up the steps—such excitement and joy—but that is the conclusion of my memory. There is no memory of arriving at the top of those steps.

I do not remember when the memory began; it has always been with me. There does not seem to be a starting point for it. The biblical similarities are those of a supreme being, omnipotent—and such love, joy and happiness in the presence of this being. Other similarities seem to be aspects of another dimension, difficult for us to understand, such as eternity (time standing still, yet passing very quickly); being able to see, but having no eyes; being able to hear, but having no ears.

As for telling anyone...I never told anyone until I was about twenty-five years old.

Francine Isom: Love that permeated the universe

Before I was born, I was allowed to remember only enough to know, without the least doubt, that we exist in a non-physical existence in a place that is indescribably loving and waiting for our return.

Let me tell you just a little about me. I'm 47, and live in Southern California. I am married almost thirty years now and have two living children and one who passed in 1992. I have always felt a closeness with the creator and have had many spiritual experiences during my life. Although I don't fully understand, I am aware that there is a great master plan, yet each of us is precious and important to the creator.

I will try to explain (within the limitations of the words we have to use) what I remember about the place I was before I was born. I have always had this memory, and asked my mother and religious leaders in my life about it, but no one could give me an answer as to what the memory was. Here is what I remember.

I am...

For what seems like forever, I am only aware that I am.

I feel nothing physical—no sense of breathing, no gravity, no senses of touch, smell, sight.

I only exist in consciousness and my consciousness is only aware that I am.

As if suspended in space—or in a void would be more accurate. There is nothing—no thought other than…I am.

My awareness perceives that I am and that I have existed for a very long time—years, possibly forever.

After this awareness has existed for quite some time, an outside thought speaks to my consciousness saying, "Remember everything. It is very important. Take in this experience. Remember every detail. It is very important."

Then my own consciousness heightens from the basic sensation of existence to an awareness that there is an environment that surrounds me that I cannot see. I perceive other people and activity but cannot see (or perhaps cannot remember the exact details). It was as if I was in a room filled with people but my eyes were shut and I couldn't open them. What I could sense was deep and complete peace, contentment and indescribable love that permeated the universe.

I strained to soak in the feeling. I spent a lot of time perceiving that existence. The outside consciousness spoke to me several times repeating what was said before, "Remember this place. It is very important. Remember everything about it."

Then, after a very long time, there was a short period of time when I was not perceiving my environment—a blank spot you might say. Then I began to get glimpses of light. First like little flashes. Then like when someone opens a door into a darkened room letting in a little light—just enough to see outlines and shadows. Gradually the light increased and I started having memories of events in my childhood, such as when I was three living in Hawaii and there was a flood and we had to sit on the top bunk bed. I have vivid memories of living in Hawaii at that age, and all through that time I would have the outside consciousness remind me to "Remember that place. Remember everything about it. It is very important to remember that place."

Between the ages of three and eight years of age, I would practice remembering. At night before I went to sleep the voice would remind me and I would go over it in my mind. I remember walking to school when I was in sixth grade and stopping dead in my tracks when the voice reminded me to "Remember that place. It is very important to remember that place." As I grew up, at about ten years old, the voice told me that I would be getting busy with my life and forget to remember the place, but I should try whenever I thought of it. This is what happened. For many years I didn't think of it, and even now I can't remember it as clearly as I did when I was five or six. I feel a little loss of the clarity of the memory, but a great sense of peace and happiness when I do think of it.

The one thing that has always puzzled me is that my child-like reasoning told me that the voice must have been God telling me to remember the place, and I thought of God as being male, yet the voice was very definitely female, kind, gentle and loving.

I believe that I was given the gift of remembrance of my pre-existence. It was as if my pre-mortal mother was preparing me for a journey and, to be sure there was no mistake or confusion, gave me the one thing that would be sure to bring me back to her—the memory of pre-existence.[2]

3

Pre-Conception Visits

When you visit the soul world through memory stories, you can almost feel yourself expanding to the stars. You might need to take a breath and breathe yourself back into the boundaried world, feel your feet touching down into three dimensions.

Since I first began gathering stories of pre-birth communication, there's been a curious progression. At first the stories I received were almost always of contacts in pregnancy. Of course the subject was new and people were shy and cautious about what they dared to share. At least in pregnancy there's some basis, a toehold in the material world. You can believe communion could happen, without having to imagine the unborn soul dancing in deep space. Almost as though our minds were being gently stretched, the balance of stories soon shifted until now (and certainly in this book) the spotlight is on the unconceived soul and its mysterious world.

Some of the clearest and most compelling pre-birth communications are those that happen before conception. Typically they come in dreams or in visions at the edge of sleep, but the soul has a rich array of techniques for getting the attention of potential parents. In stories throughout the book, we'll see many ways, such as meetings in meditation, a hovering presence, an inner voice, even messages through material objects (a falling tile, an eccentric balloon).

In these dreams and visitations, the soul often appears as a three-year-old or as an older child of perhaps six or seven. Some contacts are one-time-only. They bring an unforgettable glimpse of a child, along with the assurance that in time, we will be together.

Priscilla Tripi: "I'm waiting for you"

I had been told that I would probably never have children, and I had given up on the idea. I wasn't even thinking about having children—when I had the dream.

It was so vividly real. I remember that I was walking up a beautiful green field. At the top of the hill was a faded old farmhouse. As I got closer to the house, a little girl started to walk down the hill to meet me halfway.

I was concerned because here we were in what seemed like the middle of nowhere and this little girl was all alone. We met and she took my hand and looked up at me and I looked down at her. I asked her where her mother was and whose little girl she was. She replied, "I'm your little girl, Mommy, and I'm waiting for you."

I was just blown away! I thought, "This really is a dream, I can't have children." But a few years later, my daughter was born—and yes, the girl in the dream did look like her. The dream was about ten years ago, and now I not only have one beautiful girl but two beautiful girls.

Linda, an Englishwoman, had a glimpse of her future daughter when she herself was only eighteen years old. Her dream was like a visit to the world of souls, and curiously enough, Linda was aware that she didn't really belong there among those waiting to be born.

Linda: "You're my momma!"

Looking through your website and reading the letters, I am sitting here with my heart thumping away at the surprise that I am not the only person to have had this happen!

I had a dream that I was walking towards a large set of glass doors. The area in front of the doors was light and airy, and as I walked up to the glass doors wondering what they were there for, I noticed that beyond them was mist swirling around, and beyond the mist was another set of large glass doors.

I stood there for a while and then saw a young woman walking towards me. She was looking at me very closely, peering with a frown on her face—the kind of frown you see when someone isn't sure about something—as if to say, "Is that you? Are you who I think you are?" She then recognized me and said, "You're my momma." She was really pleased to see me! (I am English and you probably know that English children don't call their mothers "momma"!)

This young woman had blond hair and was a little shorter than me, as if she wasn't fully matured, maybe late teens. I remember thinking in the dream that this couldn't be my daughter, first because she called me "momma" and no child of mine would do that—they would call me "mum" or "mummy." And secondly, I thought that as I and my whole family are very dark-haired, and I am not attracted to blond men, this couldn't be my daughter.

She then beckoned to me with her finger to follow her and began to walk away towards the other set of glass doors. I went through the first set and on through the second set. She wanted to show me around the place where she lived. I followed her and noticed that she was pleased to be showing off her "momma." There were lots of people there, and I remember them all being young. I saw flowers, rocks—some of which were large with people sitting on them, lounging around and chatting. There was a feeling of contentment and I remember lots of smiles for me and for the pride with which my "daughter" showed me off and around.

The last thing I remember is that she wandered off somewhere and left me to stand around and look for a while. I wasn't annoyed at this at all. I was really happy there but I knew that I didn't belong, but only in the sense that I was different from all these people. They hadn't been born and I had; that was the difference.

I knew that this girl *was* my daughter but as she was so different from how I had imagined any child of mine would be, I was bemused and surprised—but really pleased, as I thought she was a pretty little thing.

I remember feeling so happy that she had shown herself to me, especially as I had quite a hard time growing up and it was like a little message of hope and happiness to help me along when I needed it. I wasn't planning on kids at the time, as I was preparing for university and travel. I didn't feel any urgency with the dream; she wasn't saying, "Have me now." She was just saying, "Hello—this is what you have to look forward to!"

When I was twenty, I met an American while in Germany. We married and had a little blond daughter called Leah! Yes, she eventually called me "momma" for a while when she was smaller (we now live in England and she has called me "mum" since she was about two years old). As for Leah—yes it is her! The face is hers, without a doubt, just older with shorter hair. The hair of the girl in my dream was a darker blond than Leah's, but her hair is getting darker as she gets older. There has never been any doubt in my mind that it was her; I knew it the moment she was born. I had the dream four years before she was born and she is now six and a total darling.

It was a lovely thing to happen and reinforced something my Dad has said to me many times over the years: that he believes we choose our parents. I knew that this little spirit had already chosen me and was waiting patiently for her birth when I was ready.

Some people experience more than just one glimpse of their child-to-be. They enjoy a series of contacts in recurring dreams or visitations, getting acquainted with their future child even before conception.

Joy H.: Falling in love with a dream child

About a year ago, I began having dreams about my son-to-be (or who I presume to be a boy). My first dream was extremely vivid. I had a beautiful baby boy, with blond curly hair and big, bright blue eyes. He grew very fast in the dream. After rafting and laughing together down a fierce river, we came to a huge, open playroom filled with games. By this point, he was about three years old, and we decided to play chess. He had extensive language skills and won the game by a long shot! I couldn't stop thinking about how proud I was to have him in my life.

Several dreams followed and included this same blond headed, vibrant little one with whom I simply fell in love. One dream consisted of just holding his hand as we traveled up an escalator. He was about four. Others have been just taking one look at him and waking up.

In February of this year, about two months after the dreams stopped, I found out that I was pregnant. Now my dreams are very vivid, yet I am simply pregnant in all of them. No sign from the little joy. Maybe it's because he is with me all the time now, in the flesh.

This is my first child and I do not know if it is a boy or a girl. I have chosen not to find out until s/he is born, yet I think I already know it is a boy! I feel quite sure, but that certainty could simply come from the dreams. (*Some time later, Joy announced that her baby was indeed a boy.*)

Renee Stock: *The little girl in my dreams*

My dreams about Mikayla started about one year before we conceived. My husband and I weren't trying to have a baby, but thought that if it happened it was meant to be. I remember going to bed one night wondering when I would become a mother. That night, I had a dream that seemed to last all night long. I was talking to a little girl in the dream. We were just light and carefree and chatting about anything and everything. I woke up remembering the dream vividly and feeling great.

Over the course of the next year, I would have a dream like this at least once a month, sometimes more often than that. We'd spend hours playing and laughing and enjoying each other. For a while I didn't know her name or even that she was the child I would give birth to. I finally asked her if she was my daughter and she said, "Yes." I asked her when I would get to meet her in the flesh and she said, "Soon." I remember asking her name, but I don't remember exactly what the first name was other than it started with an M, and the middle name was Carole after my own mother. It so happened that our favorite names started with an M: Megan, Melissa, and of course Mikayla.

Work got extremely busy the next summer and I was working what seemed like around the clock. Since I was working so hard and was so worn out, I didn't notice that my dreams of the little girl had stopped. Just when the hard push was over, I was talking to my friend's five-year-old daughter Rachael. All of a sudden, she said, "Renee, you're pregnant!" and got so excited for me. I didn't take her seriously; I didn't think it was possible. Sure enough, a week or two later, I found out that I was pregnant! When Rachael told me, I was five weeks along.

I will never forget the little girl in my dreams. My daughter has changed my life in so many ways. I've always been open to reincarnation, spiritual beings, and so on, but to have the dreams and then to see our daughter in flesh and blood...what an experience!

Not all the stories are from women, but most of them are. Does it have to be this way? In at least one traditional society, the Australian Aborigine, it is the future father who is expected to receive first contact with a child-soul. During pregnancy, a woman has a unique bond with her baby, and the physical changes can make her extra sensitive. But before conception, contact may be equally possible for either parent-to-be. A future father is sometimes the first or even the only one to sense communication, yet we seldom hear their stories. Our society doesn't encourage men to acknowledge such intimate, mysterious events.

David Brunner:[1] A Father's Visions

Beginning in 1982, I was visited on many occasions by the spirits of a young boy and girl. Though they were related, they usually came to me separately. Their names were Daniel, who appeared to be around the age of seven, and Amy, who looked to be about eight or nine years old.

Amy often gave me words of encouragement about ideas that I had. One example was when I had become stressed out and thought it would be good to get up earlier in the morning and take a walk to help get rid of the stress. It was only a passing thought till she interrupted it with her kind words, which made it seem like the best idea I'd had in a while.

The visits from Amy and Daniel were mostly inner impressions, inner voices-visions, but there was at least one time where I saw each of them appear separately (three dimensional etheric-like). One time that I saw Daniel, before he was conceived, was when I was working outside around the house. He suddenly appeared before me wearing worn, torn jeans and shirt. He repeated the words, "Need more love." Later I realized he was showing and telling me that my wife and I needed more love in our relationship; it was affecting him too.

In November of 1986 I had a dream where I heard a man's voice say, "The children are on their way down." Nine months later I was the happy father of a newborn son. When Daniel was seven, he looked just the way he had appeared to me years before he incarnated.

For Amy, it was not her time to incarnate. One of the last times I recall seeing her was when Daniel was between one and two years old. My wife and Daniel and I had just entered an amusement park. I had walked ahead of them and turned to look back with concern that Daniel, being sensitive to noise and energies, would not have a pleasant experience. Amy was standing next to Daniel, keeping him company as an older sister would.

Over the years my contact with Amy has become distant since we have moved on in our lives, but while I was writing this, she came to me with a smile, a loving heart and these kind words: "All is well…that's me, Daddy."

4

Windows on Pre-Existence

o o o o o o o o o o o o o o o o o o o o o o o o o o o o o o o

At the bottom of a very deep well,
or end of a long dark tunnel,
shimmer the glimpses of a panorama
that awaken ancient memories,
memories of the spirit's home...

Where do they live, these unborn souls who visit our dreams? Do we
have our own memories of their world? We might assume that such
memories, if they exist in us, must be deeply buried and unavailable.
Not so, according to Jerry Bongard, author of *The Near Birth Experience: Journey to the Center of Self.* In his counseling practice, Bongard
has found soul memory surprisingly easy to access.

As director of the Chrysalis Counseling Center in Bellevue, Washington, Jerry Bongard saw many clients suffering from post-traumatic
stress disorder. He found that they were helped by regressing in light
hypnosis to a time before their traumatic experiences, all the way back
to the security of the womb. But some people spontaneously went further, and re-experienced a time before being in the womb: a time
before this life. Says Bongard:

"They are invariably surprised to discover that they do not have a
body during this time before entering the womb. They may experience
the presence of other out-of-body people whom they recognize as

friends, either from this life or a previous one. They may remember speaking with these friends about the journey they are about to take into this world." As in many reports of near-death visions, they often encounter a Light that they identify as a divine being.

The experience can bring healing insight, as one relives a moment of choosing or accepting the life to come. One young man, tormented about his childhood failure to protect a sister from their father's abuse, found himself out of the body and above it, looking down at his mother from a great distance. He reported, "I can see my mother, and I can see the history of both my mother and father. It's like the DNA that goes back for hundreds of years. The strands of abuse and neglect are woven together. I know that somehow it is my job to break into that DNA and change it, to interrupt it so that my children and the next generation will not have to suffer the same kind of abuse that the previous generations had."

Imagination gives a glimpse

Soul memory is not limited to a few gifted individuals; it exists in all of us, and reveals its presence in many ways. Through imagination, dreams, poetry, and other art forms, we discover images within us that are reminiscent of soul memory.

Growing up Catholic, I learned in some detail about afterlife destinations such as Limbo, Purgatory, Hell, and Heaven. (I remember picturing the soul as a small rosy heart sailing upward, trailing a sky-blue sash.) But nothing was ever said of the soul's experience before coming into this life. Did we flash into being at the moment of conception? Without traditional teachings to guide imagination, the "before" was a gray blank.

When I was thirteen, my grandmother died—my first experience of death in the family. She gave me an unforgettable sign of her continuing existence (a story that I'll tell in a later chapter). As I followed her with my thoughts into the unknown, images arose that were strangely familiar, and I described them in poem form:

...and my soul remembering cries
O death I know you
I have died a thousand times
a thousand times have breathed again
the dark air of my unknown origin
My life leans back into slow flowing seas
my life ebbs out into the barren stars
I am as old as death...

The mind that creates poetry seems to draw from the well of soul memory. Canadian writer Silvan Waffle is the father of two girls; he and his wife also experienced a miscarried pregnancy. He muses upon the mystery of conception in his poem "Made in Secret."[1] Although he begins at the material storehouses of sperm and ova, imagination carries him somewhere quite different:

They line up
little people yet to be.
Unborn faces in a crowd of futures.
None of them exist apart from a miracle
and yet how does that make them
so different from me?
They are all in halves right now.
A few dozen in her, determined.
Many millions inside of me
still fracturing in multitudes of possibilities...
Yet now I can't help picturing them
all in a line waiting
in some shadowy star-shined
vestibule in space
pacing quietly, slowly
maybe hoping
praying
that we will seek them...

In the arts and the media there are images that take hold upon our imagination, and we discover hints of soul memory in them. To take a personal example, I suspect that "Star Trek: The Next Generation" has been so popular in part because it speaks to our hidden prenatal memories. It takes us to a place where the usual time and space constraints simply don't exist, and out into the comforting deep blue-black of space. We respond emotionally to the freedom of voyaging among the stars, while the great vessel, warm and secure, is like a bubble of light or a womb traveling through the dark. Even the harmonious society that the series portrays so well may hark back to the soul world. Do these images appeal to us because they are intimately familiar and nostalgic?

Soul Memory in Dreams

In our dreams we sometimes find ourselves in a bodiless state that seems perfectly natural and congenial to the spirit. This poem is the exact record of such a dream. At first I was puzzled by the delicious homey feel of this state, until I realized how closely it echoes soul memory stories.

> "Death is a holiday for the soul" I said
> to someone in another dream, who laughed.
> This wasn't death; so what was I doing,
>
> climbing an invisible stairway
> with no body, only my bare feet
> placing themselves higher and
>
> higher in cloudy and sky-blue space
> while a voice kept chanting "I am love, I am
> bliss, I am happiness," and happiness was
>
> natural and mine like my old blue sweater.
> Where was I going so confident,
> with no thought for the vanished planet?
>
> I might have been a christmas child
> in an advent-calendar heaven
> placing my foot higher on emptiness

and every step my step invented
glittered a moment with gold spangles,
and the silent hum suffused my

intangible body, "I am life, I am bliss,
I am happiness," and happiness was
simple and familiar as the taste of tea.

Shining through Soul Communication

Pre-birth communications can be windows to the soul world. In these experiences, we glimpse many of the same qualities that people describe when remembering pre-existence. Uplifted feelings of love, joy, peace, even humor and merriment often accompany contact with the unborn souls, as if shining around them from the "place" where they are.

A sixty-year-old woman living in Texas reminisced with me about an experience from her twenties:

> One sunny Sunday afternoon, my husband and I had been lying in bed kissing, playing, reading, talking. Eventually, I decided I needed to get up. I was just putting my feet to the floor when this light, joyous feeling swept by me (or through me) and immediately raised my spirits. The feeling came first, I believe, but I also looked up at that moment and saw a cluster of cherubs laughing down at us. I was astonished and asked my husband, do you feel that! do you see that! but he did not seem to have seen anything.
>
> What I truly remember is the lift and change and a sense of the air opening, up and to the right over my head, and an impression of merriment and children's faces laughing down. But not real children. These spirits were youthful in appearance but not in fact. Now that I've had more direct experience of *the* spirit, in visions and in the faces of other human beings, that particular elevating kind of humorous fellowship is familiar.

Theresa Danna is one of the pioneers in the field of pre-birth communication. Her interest was sparked initially by a vision of her future son, a vision that inspired Theresa's dauntless quest to bring this child into the world. But she perceived more than the beautiful little boy; she gazed through his presence into another dimension:

> One night as I was falling asleep, when I was in that half-awake/ half-asleep hypnagogic state, there appeared before my closed eyes the close-up of a toddler boy's face. At first he was looking down as if he was shy, then he slowly raised his eyes, looked directly at me, smiled, and said in his sweet voice: "Mommy, I'm coming." His eyes were the same color brown as mine, and he looked a lot like I did when I was three years old.
>
> I looked deeply into his eyes, so deeply that I was able to see beyond them. And what I saw was breath-taking. There was a bright white light and I felt pure, unconditional love pouring into me. I sensed that I was looking at eternity.
>
> While in the midst of this beauty, the impact of this child's words struck me. I'm going to be a mother! So I asked him tele- pathically, "When are you coming?" The white light went away, as well as the boy's face, and I saw the number 97. I assumed that meant my son would come to me in 1997.
>
> Then I awoke and cried tears of joy.

Three years later, in the autumn of 1997, Theresa conceived her dark-haired, brown-eyed son.

5

Conception: Energy Encounters

Among the countless books proposing to guide us through pregnancy, *The Mother-To-Be's Dream Book* is unique. Unlike most authorities, Raïna Paris boldly proposes that some of a woman's dreams in pregnancy are communications from the baby. She goes even further, acknowledging that souls may actually exist before conception. In one story from the book, a father relates an experience (not a dream) that led him to believe his child participated in her own conception:

> I am in the middle of making love to my partner, when suddenly I feel something behind me, a presence, a very powerful force, pushing my back. It is as if I am not in charge of this lovemaking any more. Someone or something has its own agenda and is using me. I was overcome with this knowing right then, like an inescapable feeling, that I had created a child, or rather that a being had used me to enter into my partner's body.[1]

We haven't studied pre-birth communication long enough to define its forms and phases in detail, but we can sketch some tentative patterns. There are typical features in experiences around the time of conception. Like the father in the story above, many parents describe an energy or a force attending them. It may feel like an impersonal presence, or give the impression of emotional qualities such as love or a sense of urgency.

A mother from the Philippines recalls: "I was a little startled to feel a presence to my left, so I turned to look. It seemed someone was there who was impatient and wanted us to 'get on with it.' It was a strong but gentle presence that hovered near the window. When I closed my eyes I could not actually see it but I knew it was there. I was sure of the time of conception, because the presence seemed to show some sense of relief soon after."

Sabrina Shane experienced an energy encounter so compelling that she recorded it before she knew whether or not it signaled conception:

Sabrina: An energy that felt alive

> We have been trying to get pregnant now for a number of months, without success. A few nights ago, I had an unusual experience. I was awakened in the middle of the night by a strong sensation of what I can only describe as a new consciousness in our home, in fact entering me and entering our combined energy—my husband's, my son's and my own.
>
> It was like there was a presence in the room, an energy that felt alive and vibrant and aware. At first I was startled, but then felt recognition. With that sensation, I experienced some sort of light. I woke my husband and told him, "I think I'm pregnant now," and related the experience to him. I'm convinced at a deep level that I had some kind of communication with our baby to be. I feel as if I was allowed to witness an entrance into this Life. It was a little unnerving but exhilarating at the same time. I'll find out soon enough if this new consciousness decided to manifest in this cycle.

Later, Sabrina confirmed that she did indeed conceive on or around that date. In her account, Sabrina mentions "some sort of light" and this too is a typical feature. Besides the encounter with an energy, people often experience an inner or outer light around conception:

Noa Bareket: A white light

I always knew immediately that I had conceived. With my first boy, I remember a kind of happiness that came after making love, and a few days later I dreamed I had a boy named Daniel. With my second boy, I felt during lovemaking that my heart opened and I loved everybody. I remember I lay in bed feeling that energy of love opening every cell in my body, and a white light that came in to me. It was beautiful.

Laura Shanley: A brilliant blue spark

My first contact with my son John came on the night of his conception. After making love, I fell asleep and had what I hesitate to call a dream, because it was so real. In the experience, I was holding the palms of my hands almost together. There was about an inch of space separating them. In that space I felt some sort of energy. I felt as if I were molding it like invisible clay. Suddenly a brilliant, blue spark appeared between my hands. I woke up and said to my husband, "I feel like I just created something!" I then went back to sleep and dreamed I was carrying around three little babies who were as big as my thumb. I loved them all dearly.

I was totally unaware of my cycles in those days, and it didn't occur to me that I had just conceived. But later, after taking a pregnancy test, I discovered that I must have conceived the night of November 30. Out of curiosity I looked in my dream journal and discovered that November 30 was the night I had those dreams.

During my pregnancy I dreamed of John several times. In most of the dreams he was floating down to me in a blue balloon, exactly the color of the spark I had seen on the night of his conception. I've gone on to have four more babies, but I never dreamed of the spark again. Nor did I ever dream of seeing my babies in a blue balloon.

But a week before John went to college, I dreamed that I saw a child sitting in a basket under a blue hot air balloon. I was standing next to the basket holding onto it, and I knew the child was mine. The balloon began to rise and I continued to hold onto it as my feet lifted off the ground. I heard a voice say to me, "It's time to let go." I let go and gently floated to the ground as the balloon and the child floated away.

Leigh Jarvis: I began to feel...electrified

My son Greg is almost eight. I had no pre-conception contact with him but I felt his soul enter my body at the moment of conception. My husband and I were at a baseball game when out of nowhere I began to feel shaky, nervous, and quite frankly electrified. My face flushed and I sensed a trembling sensation throughout my body.

It was something akin to the feelings you have when you first fall in love but much stronger. At first I thought I must be having a heart attack. It took about fifteen seconds for my mind to realize what my body already knew—I was pregnant. I'm convinced that this is the moment the sperm found the egg! My husband looked over at me to speak but stopped short; even he noticed something different! He said, "What's wrong?" I was afraid he would think I was losing it if I told him I'd just felt our child enter my body, so I said, "Nothing."

When Greg was born I "recognized" him immediately. I thought, "Of course! It's you."

From the other side: Soul memory of conception

What does the unborn soul experience at the threshold of conception? Pre-existence memories often bypass these moments, but a remarkable story from Reverend Linda Bedre[2] offers a glimpse. A counseling client (we'll call her Gwen) had a lifelong vision of her parents in a mountain cabin. In this memory-vision, Gwen sees herself floating and looking down, feeling warm and loving and excited. When Rev. Bedre encouraged her to explore the vision and to expand what she thought it was about, Gwen came up with a creation story.

She next asked her mother about the cabin, describing it in detail inside and out, colors and all. Her mother gasped, for she and her fiancé had gone to a friend's cabin a week before the wedding and had made love for the first time in their relationship. Feeling ashamed, they

3

Conception: Energy Encounters33

never talked about having been there, and Gwen had always been told in a joking way that she had been conceived on the wedding night. Her mother was amazed at the accuracy of Gwen's report.

From Brazil comes an almost poetic soul memory. Retired engineer Armando Vettorazzo says, "I am not a professional in this area, but deeply interested in the mysteries of life." While undergoing a form of regression therapy developed by Brazilian psychologist Renate Jost de Moraes, Mr. Vettorazzo found himself experiencing the moments before conception.

Armando: Flooded with Living Light

In one of the sessions, I saw my father in an armchair reading a newspaper, and at the same time I saw my mother near the stove in the kitchen. This scene reappeared several times; eventually the therapist agreed I should examine it more closely.

In that scene, I perceived myself as a simple point floating in space. I could see both my father and my mother even though there were walls between her and myself. My father called her and she left what she was doing and approached him. He showed her a recipe for a certain dish that he had found in the newspaper and wanted her to prepare. There was a clear sense of his scorn for my mother's cooking. That recipe in the paper—yes, it must be much better than hers. His manner was fairly rude. I felt her annoyance, and that she was hurt by the way her husband treated her. She answered him rather sharply; the hostile climate between them was clear to me.

At that moment I noticed the presence of a light, to my left and a little above me. I had the feeling that I had come from that light. From that moment on, the light grew more intense, enveloping my parents, illuminating them and making them shine. The atmosphere between them changed immediately. My father got up, and they stood facing each other and looking into each other's eyes. I perceived affection and tenderness in his gaze, and tenderness and understanding in hers. I could feel the love that united them. The feelings of each were my own feelings; I was one with them both.

Then something very strange happened. Still perceiving myself as a point in space, I saw the two of them on the other side of the room, holding hands and walking toward their bedroom. I also saw something which I knew to be myself as well, like a star with five rounded points, like a thick transparent jelly, embracing their shoulders and guiding them towards the bedroom.

During the session, I would tell the therapist everything that was happening and he would ask questions to clarify the meaning of what I saw or felt. When I said I was guiding them toward the bedroom, the therapist asked, "Why are you directing them?"

I found myself saying, quite surprised that he didn't know since it seemed obvious, "Well, so they can make what I need, my body!"

In another session, I decided to ask the Wise One to show me something of my gestation. (The Wise One is an imaginary figure that supposedly knows the contents of the unconscious and acts as a device to facilitate access to it.) I saw myself as a point in space in the bedroom, observing my parents in bed where they were engaged in sex. I lived that act in its entirety with all that was felt and experienced, being alternately my father and my mother. Then I saw myself again as that same point in space observing them now lying side by side, and I perceived the presence of that light emanating love, understanding, and approval. The whole room was flooded with that living light. There was an expansive feeling of peace, harmony and sacredness. It was a holy moment, pure and sublime without any sense that sex was something to be kept hidden.

6

Announcings

There's a special delight in stories of pre-birth communications that announce a pregnancy. Sometimes these encounters come unexpectedly to people who have given up hope of ever having a child. Their cases offer poignant evidence for the reality of soul contact.

Waking visions and dreams are typical ways for the unborn soul to reveal its presence, but occasionally a pregnancy is literally announced by a voice. Mary had just asked her college instructor a question, when her hearing was somehow interrupted by an inner voice. Instead of the professor's words, she heard: "The reason you have felt physically burdened and emotionally burdened is because you have invited me into your life. I am here with you. I am here." Next day, she learned that she was two weeks pregnant.

The following stories relate announcing dreams that came when the hope of having a child was nearly gone. The first account is from Brazil.

Dayse: "She is exactly that baby from my dream"

I believe I have been waiting for my daughter all my life. I always wanted to have just one child, and that child would be a girl (at least, in my imagination there was never a boy). It seemed it was never the right time to have a baby, until I turned thirty-five and decided I should have my child. My husband didn't feel he was ready to be a father, but for me it seemed the most important thing in the whole world, this child.

How can I describe my feelings? It's like I already missed the child who wasn't born yet. I used to sit and just have that squeezing sensation in my heart, longing to see her, to be with her. I used to be sad because she wasn't with me, and my husband could not understand it. I tried to get pregnant, but for ten months nothing happened. I got to the point when I gave it up. I wasn't thinking about it any more, and I thought that maybe God didn't want me to have children.

In January, 1995, I went to bed feeling very tired—I had been feeling that way for a week—and I simply "saw" my girl. I was in a big empty room, and right there in front of me, across the room, was this baby about ten months old, dressed in white, sitting on the floor with her legs wide apart, smiling sweetly at me.

I woke up feeling strange, moved, and that sensation was with me all day long. I told this dream to my mother, who knew I'd had strange experiences with dreams before, but she didn't know what to make of it.

Guess what! That same January I went to the doctor because I felt tired all the time, and the blood test told me I was three weeks pregnant. The dream had come to me when I was one week pregnant. In spite of the dream and in spite of wanting a girl, for seven months I thought I was having a boy. When I learned it was a girl, I couldn't hold back my tears of happiness.

I used to tell my mother during my pregnancy that my baby would be warm, cheerful, calm, and very sweet. I used to say, "She will love you so much you won't believe it." My daughter was born in October, and ever since she was able to smile, she would smile preferentially to me and to my mother. She would wave her little arms, all excited, every time my mother was around.

She is exactly that baby from my dream. I recognized the white clothes one day when she was seven or eight months old and she was sitting on the floor. My mother had given them to her before she was born when we didn't know her sex. My girl has the exact personality I thought she would have. She looks at my mother's face as if she knew her more deeply than she knows any other person, including me. My Leticia came to this world to be with us again—my mother and me. I can't explain how I know this, but I just know we were meant to be together, and that I waited thirty-six years for my baby girl.

One last curious thing: When my child was about eleven months old, I asked her in my thoughts, one night while she was sleeping and I stood by her side: "Who were you, before you were born?" I went to bed and had a dreamless sleep, but my mother called me the next morning, excited and moved, to tell me she had had a marvelous dream about Leticia. In this dream, Leticia was playing quietly when she suddenly looked into my mother's eyes, smiled, and began telling her "wonderful things, with her baby voice, but with clear words which caused me to just stare at her, amazed at the things she was telling me about herself!"

Cindi: More peaceful than I had ever felt

Having experienced pre-birth communication nearly twenty-five years ago, I am amazed to find others like me. I never met anyone who could relate to my story and I felt rather alone. I honestly don't think friends believed me when I told them of it.

I had tried to get pregnant for quite some time. I had been told it was highly unlikely since I'd had a rather bad bout of endometriosis when I was nineteen. I persisted because I had this feeling—a feeling that there was a child of mine waiting to be born and that I *must* get pregnant. Everyone thought I was crazy, but I knew I must keep trying.

Then I dreamed the most vivid dream of my life, before or since. I saw myself and my then mate pushing a stroller at the top of a hill. Inside that stroller was a darling baby boy. He was blond, blue eyed, a beautiful child, and we were calling him "Zak." When I awoke from this dream, I felt more peaceful than I had ever felt and knew, without question, not only that I would become pregnant, but who the child was and how he looked, long before he was born. Within two weeks I learned that I was indeed pregnant.

Throughout my pregnancy, when people asked me whether I wanted a boy or a girl, I would tell them it wasn't a matter of what I wanted—that I already knew the little person inside me, knew it was a boy and that his name was Zak.

Nine months after the dream, my son was born. He looked precisely like the dream child, down to every detail. I knew this child completely by the time he entered the world and to this day, we share a bond so inexplicably close that we still feel as though we share the same breath and the same heartbeat. As I have aged (I'm nearly fifty now), I've come to believe that each of us has a purpose on this planet, a reason for being here. I firmly believe my reason is so that Zak could be here. I don't feel so alone with my experiences any more.

Like Cindi, the hopeful parents in the next story were driven by a mysterious conviction that, in spite of discouraging evidence to the contrary, they would have a child. Perhaps this inner assurance is another kind of telepathic communion with the unborn soul.

Jean*: The Third Dream

My husband and I suffered from infertility for eleven years. We just assumed we would have children, but they never came. We went to doctor after doctor till we eventually found one who diagnosed my husband's blockage. After unsuccessful surgery to remove the blockage, we nearly gave up, but we both knew we had to keep trying. Although on the surface we lived as if we would never have any children together, privately we knew that we would.

I was thirty-seven and my husband was forty. I prayed for help. Dave* was close to his grandfather who had passed away, so I asked this grandfather if he could pray for Dave from the other side. I know it sounds crazy but I felt compelled.

Finally we decided to try in vitro fertilization. The chance of success was only 38%, and we only had the money for one try! It didn't matter. We both *knew* we would have our son. We were told that three eggs were fertilized, a low number compared to the average. We rejoiced and Dave hoped for triplets, but I didn't feel that this would happen.

Then came the day for the implantation of the eggs. The in-vitro room was dark with a TV screen so we could watch the process. Our emotions ran high and Dave was breaking out in a sweat as he held my hand. At the moment it was done I had an incredible vision of my mother standing in the room. This was very shocking to me. Then a great peace came over me.

That night in the hotel room I had to stay in bed. I fell asleep and dreamed that I was sitting at a table with Dave and my mother. I went to the bathroom and came out crying that I lost one of my babies. My mother tried to comfort me. The next night I had a similar dream! Since I only had three eggs implanted I didn't want a third dream like that.

On the third night I dreamed that I was home. Sitting at our kitchen table with us was a little boy with bright blue eyes and fine golden brown hair like Dave's (I have thick black hair). The little boy had a glass of milk that he tipped over and spilled. I told him that if he didn't want it he just had to say so. He giggled. The next night the same boy was in my dream and he was celebrating his birthday. I gave him a big hug and we were very happy.

We had two weeks to wait before we could find out if the implantation was successful. I went to my local doctor to have a sonogram. There on the screen was a tiny heartbeat! I had one little embryo that stuck. It's hard to describe the emotions at that time. Dave was at work and I called to tell him the wonderful news. He told me that the night before he'd had a dream that his grandfather came to see him, patted him on the back and said, "Congratulations, Dave!" He said he hadn't thought about his grandfather in years. I guess my prayer was heard!

Little Paul* is now a healthy toddler with his dad's bright blue eyes and fine golden brown hair. Incidentally, since he began eating baby food, he will drink milk but it isn't his favorite. One day he was sitting in his high chair and knocked over his glass of milk and spilled it. When I frowned and went to clean it up, he started giggling.

The Child at the Foot of the Bed

Two mothers relate similar visions, but there is one illuminating difference between their circumstances: one is a birth mother, the other an adoptive mother. The first woman writes while awaiting her daughter's birth:

We have twin boys now in high school and love them very much. Yet a face was missing from our family and we tried for many years to produce a little girl. After finally accepting that another child was not in the picture for us, we decided to wait for our grandchildren to be born.

Before I knew that I was pregnant, I had a vision of a little girl bathed in a golden light at the foot of my bed. I knew she had a strong connection to me and my family and that she was wise and loving. Somehow she reached me. It was a timeless experience. From that point on, there have been many spiritual experiences—wordless communications that surround her, through dreams and thoughts and countless other ways that cannot be defined with language.

The second woman's story is told in *Coming From the Light*, by Sarah Hinze. Unable to have another child, Cheryl and her husband had tried unsuccessfully to adopt. One night, Cheryl heard a child calling her. Assuming it was one of her daughters, she raised her head to listen for the voice again, but to her surprise she saw a shadow-like figure of a child at the foot of the bed. She could make out dark hair and a dark complexion.

Thinking her eyes were playing tricks on her, Cheryl reached for her glasses, but the figure was still there, stretching out its arms toward her. She thought, "What do you want?" and the answer she heard was: "Mommy, it's time for me to come."

Encouraged by the vision, Cheryl and her husband applied again to adopt a child. After a short time (and several "coincidences" that moved their application quickly through the process), they became the parents of a Native American baby.

Although there are only a few adoption stories in this collection, they are particularly meaningful because they demonstrate that soul connections transcend biological relationships. Whether coming by birth or by adoption, the soul communicates in much the same way.

Mary Anne: Announced by joy

This experience occurred with our second child. This little daughter is adopted. We were finished with the extensive paperwork and interviews and were waiting to hear from the marvelous agency with whom we were working. In May of that year I found that whenever I rested to pray, I was filled with an awareness that our daughter was about to be born. I felt as though I was invited to be a part of this birth. Of course I prayed for her birth mother and for her well-being. I asked Jesus and His mother Mary to guide them through the birth.

I felt so full and so joyous. I can't really explain how special it was. When that month was over the awareness and the fullness left. I expected that the adoption agency would call us any day soon. Months went by and the agency never called. Gradually I set aside that experience. In March of the following year the agency called and asked us to be the parents of a little girl. When we looked at the information they had about her, I discovered that she had been born in May of the previous year.

7

Communing in Pregnancy

We might assume that the nine months of pregnancy would be the perfect, easiest time for connecting with the baby-to-be. But in fact, pregnancy is a rather complicated setting for soul communication. Now we have the awareness of being pregnant, and all our hopes, fears, wishes, and guesses about the baby are added to the mix. How can we sort out the elements of real communication—information transmitted from mind to mind? In pregnancy, the reality may be more one of communion, shared fields—a kind of psychic merging.

A mother may intuit much about her unborn child. We receive impressions from the baby's physical presence and the way it moves in the womb. (Dream researcher Robert Van de Castle, noting how reliably a pregnant woman's dreams predict her baby's sex, ponders whether there may even exist "extremely sensitive cellular receptors in the uterus" that could sense the difference between a male and a female embryo.[1]) Gathering impressions about the baby, we might present them to ourselves in a dream, dramatized as a meeting with the child.

A truly mind-boggling complicating factor, not just in pregnancy but in all pre-birth communication, is the mystery of time and the possibility of precognition. Robert Moss, author of *Dreaming True*, asserts that we all naturally and routinely dream the future, sometimes meeting people in dreams whom we won't actually encounter for years to come. A story told by Candace Pfau is a thought-provoking example. How can we explain this kind of knowing?

Candace: The horse that wasn't there

My mother dreamed of my daughter before we even knew she existed. She described my daughter in such detail that when the caseworker brought me the photo of this girl, I recognized her instantly. My husband and I were thinking about adopting a toddler, but we had been on the waiting list for a year when my mother told me about her dream. She said, "I was seeing your family, and the three boys were there, and there was a little girl with you, about eight years old with light brown hair and gray eyes and a very heart shaped face."

Then my mother added, "And there was a horse on the fence by your neighbor's house." At the time of this dream, I was wanting a little girl of about three. So I laughingly told my mother, "The neighbors do not have a horse, so no problem."

About three months later, the caseworker called and said, "I know you had your heart set on a three-year-old, but we have an eight-year-old whom we need to place right away." I asked to see a picture. When I saw the picture, that was it. About six months after our daughter came to live with us, the neighbors got a horse. So, when I first went into the adoption process, I thought I was picking out my child, but now I realize that plans were already in progress, and someone far wiser than I was placing her.

Fortunately, it isn't my goal to prove soul communication or to decide which experiences are intentional contacts from the unborn child. I believe we are souls (or perhaps one soul refracted into the appearance of many), and that as souls we are not entirely limited by time and space. We know things about each other and about our unborn children by many means, and we may not always be able to tease apart the various strands and sources of our knowing. The riddle is evident in the next two stories. Precognition—or pre-birth communication?

Sue Shephard: She showed me a piece of the future

My older sister had two boys and I felt especially close to my blond, blue-eyed nephew, being blond and blue-eyed myself. Whenever I would take him out, people assumed he was my son because of the resemblance. So when I found out I was pregnant, I just took it for granted that I'd have a little blond, blue-eyed boy. I've always known my son's name would be Michael, but never gave a girl's name any real thought. Why would I? I was going to have a boy!

One night, I dreamed I was at my mother's house. They have a narrow stone walkway and I was crouched down on the walk. This little girl of about three, all dark curls and chub, came running over to me calling, "Mommy! Mommy!" and holding out a fistful of flowers. The name "Gina" passed through my mind and then I woke up. Even after the dream, as nice as it was, I continued to assume I would have a boy.

Flash-forward about three and a half years. It's summertime and I'm at my parents' house. My daughter runs up to me calling "Mommy!" while I'm sitting on the lawn next to the stone walkway. In the dream, she was the exact image of what she was in reality at that age. The same shape of face, the same pudgy little hands, the same dark curls. It amazes me even today when I think of it. It was her! I believe she visited me while she was in my womb and showed me a piece of the future.

Christine Maraccini: That Giggle

My pregnancy was a little rough. I had terrible morning (noon, and night) sickness, and I had trouble breathing due to the baby's position. The last couple of months, I was hardly able to lie down to sleep. One evening I was completely exhausted and tired of sleeping on the chair in the living room, so I tried to lie down in our bed. To my surprise, my son had moved a bit and I wasn't as uncomfortable as usual. That night I had the most incredible dream. *(At the time of the dream, Christine knows her baby is a boy.)*

Everything was very vivid, almost real. My son was about two years old and we were sitting on the floor playing with blocks. He said, "Mommy, I'm going to build you a castle!" And then he giggled; I will never forget that giggle. He had sandy blond hair and bright blue eyes. He was a stocky little guy, sort of big for his age. He was wearing blue jeans, a little red checked flannel shirt, and brown hiking boots. My husband was sitting near us on the sofa, laughing. We played for hours, going to the park and sliding down the slide and swinging next to each other.

I woke up the next morning, very excited. I told my husband that I knew what our son was going to look like and I described him. Fortunately, my husband believes in my intuitive senses, so he was excited too.

My son is almost ten months old now. He has sandy blond hair and bright blue eyes. He is stocky and pretty big for his age. The first time I heard him giggle, I knew that I had heard that sound before, months ago when all I wanted was some encouragement and a good night's sleep.

Being Available

For some parents-to-be, it's a stretch to imagine their child existing as a soul before conception. With pregnancy and the physical reality of a fetus, making contact may seem more natural. But how do you get in touch? As one Englishwoman asked, "How can you hear what your baby is saying to you?"

The simplest suggestion is: just make yourself available. It's difficult to tune in when we're chronically distracted and hurrying through the days. Of course, pregnancy has a way of slowing us down, but there are specific things we can do to become more receptive.

About half of all communication experiences occur in altered states such as dreams, meditation, or deep relaxation. Look for the settings and situations that help you shift your focus inward, quieting the mental noise. Whether in pregnancy or before conception, people have felt the soul presence of their child while receiving a massage, taking a shower, walking in nature, chopping vegetables, washing the dishes…

The easiest way to set the stage for encountering your baby is to begin tuning in to your dreams. Thomas Verny, in *Nurturing the Unborn Child*, suggests that before going to sleep you focus upon your baby and affirm, "Tonight I will meet my unborn child in my dreams." You can invite the soul to enter your dreams, even make an appointment for a visit.

Communication can happen in many different ways. It may not be in words, though some mothers find themselves having inner conversations with their baby. Some people are especially good at visualizing, and find this is the channel they can use to reach the soul. Others may simply feel a presence and be inspired to communicate their own feelings. It's easy to overlook the unexpected forms of communion. It could be something as subtle as an unfamiliar mood, an impulse, a poem spilling itself into the heart. Sometimes it is only in looking back, years later, that we can see how unusual an experience was.

Can we feel the presence of a soul in an almost physical way? My personal answer is "Yes!" since I've twice been blessed to sense such contacts from the "dead." Melissa's experience shows that unborn souls, too, can reach across whatever separates us, and impress us with a loving touch.

Melissa: Soul Kiss

While meditating during a prenatal yoga class, I was focusing on my baby and asking her to work with me during her birth. I felt she would sense my true feelings so I let her know I was a little scared of the pain, and also of her feeling pain as she's pushed through the birth canal. Then I felt the presence of my child's soul all around me, and she kissed my cheek. I felt she was letting me know it would be all right.

It was not like the physical sensation of being kissed, yet I was aware of a loving presence right next to me. I felt surprised and comforted; I remember being very still because I was in a meditation pose, but I became tearful and shuddered a bit. I have often visualized her body within mine and of course I feel her move about, but I had not felt this presence make itself known before in a distinct spiritual way.

Pre-birth communications are similar in many ways to after-death contacts. Dream visits, waking visions, touches, lights, and sense of presence—all these are used by souls on either side of earth-life. However, there is one method that seems to be a favorite for the dead, but rare in pre-birth contacts. This is the manipulation of physical objects, especially electrical ones.

Barbara W: Light bulbs and balloons

When my daughter Jessi was one year old, I became pregnant with twins, but miscarried both within a couple of months. I experienced another miscarriage of a little girl who had trisomy-9, and one more very early miscarriage.

I was deeply saddened and discouraged. Throughout my infertility drugs and shots, and increasingly with each miscarriage, I began to resign myself to the fact that the likelihood of delivering another child was remote. However, a force kept pressing me on throughout my miscarriage-pregnancy roller coaster.

Electrical toys would turn on and off by themselves, especially a talking telephone. Whenever this occurred, I sensed a spiritual presence. Having already experienced three miscarriages, I was hesitant to hope for the best. During the pregnancy attempt in December 1996, I was thinking to myself, "I'm probably not pregnant," because I didn't want to be disappointed again. Suddenly the overhead light in my bedroom started getting dimmer and brighter, over and over again. I shut the light off and turned it back on about thirty seconds later and it did the same thing. Shortly thereafter, I had a positive pregnancy test. Ultrasound eventually confirmed a quad pregnancy, but one of the four had been miscarried.

During this successful triplet pregnancy, my daughter Jessi and I observed a Pooh balloon (which was touching the ceiling) maneuver its way around the Barney balloon, travel down the hall to the Pooh nursery, and move down a foot to the door. The door was shut, so the balloon came back down the hall and entered Jessi's bedroom. As it moved down to enter the room, the string attached to the balloon got caught on an art project that was taped to her door. The balloon tried to tug free, but it was stuck. After a couple of tugs, three of the light bulbs in a chandelier over the kitchen table simultaneously blew out, with a popping sound! Jessi and I just stared in amazement, and I felt a lot of energy.

We are often surprised to receive an unexpected contact, but we can also choose to initiate contact. Stories throughout the book show many ways of reaching toward the unborn soul and inviting communication. Shauna visualized and relaxed her way into communion with her baby:

Shauna: A visit to the womb

My second child, unlike my first, was planned and very anticipated. When I found out I was pregnant I was excited and did everything to ensure a "perfect pregnancy." I chose not to find out the sex of this child, but to be honest I really wanted a boy, as I already had a daughter.

At about ten weeks I was lying in bed, rubbing my tummy lovingly and envisioning what life would be like thirty weeks from then. Before I knew it I was talking to my belly. I relaxed and envisioned myself traveling down through my body to my womb where I "saw" my child. I perceived him as a baby in utero, not really fetal nor full term. He told me he was a boy and that he loved me. He seemed very grown up in our conversation. It was short, but I felt a strange sense of calm reassurance. I had no doubt that I was carrying a boy.

Many communications in pregnancy take the form of a simple message almost like a news bulletin, often coming in response to a parent's concern or intense curiosity. Isabelle was in early pregnancy, pondering whether her child would be a boy or girl, when she felt a powerful inner voice. It announced, "My name is Abraham, I'm a little male child; it takes nine months to make a body, then we'll meet." Her first reaction, she says, was to look skyward and think, "Oh my God, I've gone crazy," but she quickly realized that her child was communicating with her. (And yes, he was a boy!)

Sandra Greiner was curious about "who" was inside her while pregnant with her second child. One night her daughter appeared in a vivid, almost lucid dream. She looked about fifteen months old, very beautiful and with a strong resemblance to her father. She said, "Mom, I just want you to know that I am a girl and I am very healthy, so don't worry. I will look just like Dad." When the baby was born, her information proved to be accurate.

Some messages are more complex. Cassandra Eason is the English author of excellent books including *A Mother's Instincts* and *The Mother Link*. In *The Mother Link*, she presents one of the most impressive accounts of pre-birth communication on record. While pregnant, Felicity enjoyed talking to her unborn child. Gradually she became aware that she was hearing an inner response and having actual conversations. At six months pregnant, Felicity asked the baby if she was healthy and received an affirmative reply. Being an anxious first-time mother, she went on to ask if there were any blemishes on her body. "Well," the baby told her, "I do have a birthmark on my heel that is shaped like an apple." There were no such marks in the family history, but when the little girl was born, she proved to have an apple-shaped birthmark on one heel.[2]

Blending the Borders

A pregnant woman and her unborn child may be in such close psychic contact that the borders of their being almost melt into one another. From this blending, unfamiliar moods and cravings and images arise. My own cravings while pregnant with my firstborn were strange for me: snowy mountain peaks, stories of Himalayan treks, and longings for isolated communities of women.

In *The Tibetan Art of Parenting*, Anne Hubbell Maiden recounts a belief that the unborn baby's consciousness manifests in the mother's dreams. "In the Tibetan tradition, dreams are often a way for a person, or an unborn baby, to bridge life in this world with other lives…[T]he mother may experience unusual dreams, as if they belonged to somebody else. There may be different settings that seem unfamiliar, yet somehow important. A mother who attends to these dreams may have hints about her child's earlier lives and calling or the child's purpose in this life."

Jeni Lee's story of pre-birth connections with her daughter shows how dreams and other ways of communing can give us advance knowledge of the person coming to be born.

Jeni Lee: The Story of Alora

About three years ago, when I meditated I would be overwhelmed by a strong and concerned, almost desperate presence. It made me feel uncomfortable because I didn't know how to help the spirit. It began telling me, through feelings, that it had a destiny and needed my health; I heard her say, "I want to be born." I felt her presence from time to time while driving, sitting, just about anywhere, and continued to feel her pressing need in the back of my mind. I could sense her urgency and it pained me because it was not happening. I thought I was pregnant a couple of times but each time, even after having strange physical experiences, I was told no.

I remember finding out that I was pregnant and hearing her voice say, "Mommy, I want to be born this time." I dreamed that she was destined to go to (or has come from) Tibet and that I should expose her to Buddhist teachings. I love the spirit inside me, know we have met before, and that she chose me for a specific reason; I feel it is to encourage her unique spiritual gifts.

The dream about Tibet came when I was not even three months pregnant and I was resting on the couch in between bouts of all day sickness. I saw the mountains, the monasteries, the people, the animals, smelled the food and saw her in formal robes as a powerful woman preparing to wed a powerful man in hopes that they could unite a people. In that dream she was pale with dark hair. She is always tall. She is beautiful and ethereal.

I see her playing with Runes and Tarot cards. I see her being strong, unique, incredibly alive, in fairylike clothes, dancing outside of society and conventions. Alora is an old soul, older than I am. I sense she knows more and sees more. She often tells me that everything will be all right, when I get nervous or scared. She encourages me, through feeling, to continue my spiritual quest. She talks to me when I think to her and we are always explaining things to each other. The other night something told me to put my hand on my belly where she was and I felt a flow of love energy traveling between us, and heard the words and felt them, "I love you."

I mostly interact with her telepathically, in hopes we will be able to keep that going after birth, as my mother and her grandmother did; they could talk without words over great distances. I also talk to her verbally and through touch. I teach her letters, numbers, words, shapes, sounds, smells, and play music. When her dad talks to her or reads to her she just loves it, she feels all warm and happy, moves toward his voice and starts playing. She is an incredible person, already so influential in our lives, and she has definitely chosen us. I have no doubt about that!

My mother has visited with her many times. She has quite a time catching up with her—Alora seems to be in constant motion. Mom also sees her playing with Runes and Tarot cards and feeling frustrated that many people do not understand her or her destiny. Like me, she senses that Alora is feeling urgency in her destiny to help a large group of people reunite or find peace. She senses too that Alora has chosen us to help her get where she needs to be, since we understand. We will work to maintain a telepathic bond with her, long after she is born.

Jeni Lee adds, "By the way, Alora was re-born to this plane on June 24, 2000—she is perfect!"

8

Outside Connections

o o o o o o o o o o o o o o o o o o o o o o o o o o o o o o

The day I found out I was pregnant, my best friend called me…She had a dream so vivid that she felt like my baby boy (boy!) had called her on the phone to announce his presence, his sex, his appearance (blue eyes, wavy reddish hair), and his name.

—*Anne*

Although it's often said that we are all psychic, the truth seems to be that we vary in our ability to receive and recognize telepathic messages. And so, as dream explorer Robert Moss affirms, the unborn child communicates not only with its parents, but with other receptive people in the environment who may find themselves enlisted as go-betweens.[1]

Moss calls these people "soul-helpers," and the information they receive is often about a needed change to help the mother or the growing baby, such as adding more protein to the mother's diet. But sometimes the message is more like a happy announcement, as if the soul is introducing itself to a third person who will repeat the news aloud to the parents. It reminds me of the old-fashioned custom of sending a singing telegram—a way of adding oomph to the greeting! Then too, by interacting with someone independent of any physical connection, the soul adds weight to the evidence that it exists and can communicate.

In the following story, there is no obvious deep connection between the unborn child and the person who received its message. Susan and Kay* were simply co-workers throughout Kay's pregnancy. The physical closeness, and the fact that Susan is an empathetic person, seem to have helped her form a telepathic link with Kay's baby.

Susan: A message from the baby

Kay was due in about three weeks. We weren't especially close but we chatted often at work. One Friday, Kay was on her way out the door and called back to me that she'd see me on Monday. I blurted out, "No, you won't, you're having your baby on Sunday." It somewhat shocked both of us to hear those words come out, but we shrugged it off and she said, "I wish."

On Sunday night, I had a very disturbing dream about Kay. She was standing alone in a dark room with her arms wrapped around herself, weeping. Through the doorway I could see a bassinet with a light shining on it. I knew this was her newborn and that he was very sick with something life-threatening. Kay had never mentioned any problems with the baby, so I knew this was a surprise. During the dream, however, I felt compassion for Kay but I knew everything was fine. I knew they both had a difficult road but that everything would be just fine—and this was a message from the baby.

When I got to work that morning, I learned that Kay had her baby son on Sunday and he was born with several holes in his heart. Kay came into the office about a month later so I took that opportunity to tell her about my dream, hoping it would give her some comfort. She looked at me like I was crazy and burst into tears, so I don't think I helped.

Three years later, after several surgeries, Kay's little boy is fine and healthy. I've often wondered why I was given this glimpse into their personal lives. I imagine the baby was trying to tell "someone" that he would be all right, and Kay was too distraught to take comfort.

As Susan observes, the person who is most emotionally involved may not be able to recognize a message as easily as can an outside observer. On two occasions in my days as a yoga teacher, I received crystal-clear impressions of the sex of a student's unborn child, but with my own babies I was much less sure. While I cared about my students, I wasn't really curious to know their babies' sex, so the information could appear in my thoughts like an unmistakable island in a calm sea. A soul trying to communicate some news about itself may sometimes find it easier to deal with a neutral outsider than to cut through the many ideas in its own parent's mind.

A Gift for Birth Attendants

Claire Winstone, a student of perinatal psychology, asks: "Have you heard any stories of communication from babies during the time of birth?" Claire goes on to explain that in recalling her own birth she realized there had been no one present who was aware of what she was experiencing. "I felt that everyone was out of sync with me—variously coaching impatiently, and panicking, when in my own pain and terror I most needed connection and gentle, sensitive reassurance and encouragement that I could survive that last agonizing scrape over the sacrum and ischial spines."

The unborn soul's ability to communicate does open up wondrous possibilities for easing the transition of birth. It is exciting to learn that some babies and birth attendants, like Joy in the following story, have discovered how to use telepathic communication to help one another in pregnancy and labor.

Joy*: The babies talk to me

I am a nurse-midwife in private practice. Occasionally an unborn baby of one of my patients "talks" to me telepathically. Most often this happens during labor to suggest some position change to make descent easier, or to tell me of a change in maternal blood pressure, maternal fever, and so on. This information always proves true and often shortens labor.

Sometimes the "talking" happens during prenatal office visits to tell me of something affecting the mother at home that I wouldn't otherwise know, such as drug abuse, domestic violence, or extreme stress. I use the information to bring up the subject nonchalantly with the mother and we talk about options from there. These communications do not happen with every baby, seem to be for specific purposes, and end abruptly with the delivery of the baby's head (almost as if it has passed through some veil and communication is not possible for me now).

At least three times I have heard a joyful "I'm coming! I'm coming right now!" as the baby makes a rapid descent and precipitous delivery. I am rushing to the bedside fumbling with my gloves. I ask the baby, "Would you please wait until I get my gloves on?" The reply is always the same: "I can't. I've got to come right NOW!" I know the mothers and fathers must wonder why their nurse-midwife is bursting out laughing as their little one is entering the world, but I get tickled at the baby's excited comments and insistence on rushing right out!

All the weird things in my life started when I was a child and I saw colors around everyone, saw spirits and my "pretend" playmate. I thought everyone had these experiences until I mentioned them casually to my mama one day around the age of eight. She abruptly told me I was seeing things or making up a story. I tried again at the age of twelve to tell her about what I saw and got the same reaction. So I learned never to speak of it again.

By the way, both of my daughters are showing some indications of intuitive behaviors. I am not discouraging this in any way, unlike my mama. I ask them to tell me everything they see and to draw pictures for me. I do not want to feed overactive imaginations, but to support future seers and hearers! I have told them that although none of this is bad, and in fact it is a gift from God that Mama sees things and hears things, we shouldn't go around telling everyone, because so many folks do not understand.

The "talking babies" started about ten years ago after graduation from midwifery school, not during my earlier work as a labor and delivery nurse. I just thought it was another of those strange things that I needed to keep to myself and not share with anyone. Last fall I blurted out to a counselor about seeing the colors and how they upset me sometimes, and she referred me to a wonderful person who does energy work. I now understand that I see auras (duh!) and am learning something like Therapeutic Touch to use the gift to help others.

I am filled with joy to discover that there are others who experience similar things! I would love to share more stories with you in hopes of someone else learning that they are not crazy.

Joy's next story, about communicating with baby Kevin, is magical. This unborn soul communicated not only words and ideas but waves of emotion. At first, Joy may have been just a conveniently receptive outsider, but her conversations with Kevin created a deep soul friendship.

"The most intense feelings I have ever experienced"

It all started with a terrifying call from my friend's mother: "We just found out Lynn* was raped several months ago, and she is pregnant—pretty far along. Will you come over right now?" You can imagine the genuine shock we all felt—including the birth mother. She had been in deep denial about the assault and the pregnancy. Even though she was six months along, she hadn't allowed herself to accept it until the doctor's visit that day proved the pregnancy.

This shows one of my "blind spots." I am sure all of us who see and hear things must have blind spots, and it is important to know what yours are! I am not one of those people who can just look at a woman and say "you're pregnant" long before she knows or shows. We all probably know some wise old woman who has this ability. But I cannot know a woman is pregnant until she knows and accepts it. Often then I can know the sex of the baby.

Up until this time, I had only short, specifically purposeful communications with a few babies of my patients—approximately three or four a month. But that night started a long-term, frequent connection between Lynn's baby and me. He started talking to me that night very soon after I arrived at her mother's home.

I knew the baby was a boy. He expressed disappointment that his hiding place had been found out. It was almost like a little boy with a secret tree house that has just been discovered by adults. He knew he would be discovered at some point, but he was "bummed out!" He said his mother knew about him, of course, on some unconscious level, and that the family dog had known about him from almost the beginning. But he was terrified by the family reaction to his presence. He kept saying over and over, "Don't let them hurt me...Please don't let them hurt me."

As a nurse-midwife, I was the immediate objective consultant who laid out all the options for my friend. She was about to start the last possible week where termination was legal in our state. As much as I disliked that option this late in pregnancy and as hard as it was to discuss above the roaring comments by the baby, I still presented all options to Lynn in a nonbiased fashion. This was her decision to make. After several days she chose adoption as the option she wanted. We all agreed to support her in any decision, but the baby expressed relief to me with this one.

Throughout her pregnancy he continued to talk to me, frequently at times, and then not for days at other times. He explained that it didn't matter to him how he was conceived but that he was coming for a purpose. I asked him which he would choose, if given a choice between being raised by his biological mother or being adopted. His answer consistently was, "I will be where I am supposed to be." He seemed to be a wise, older presence, always answering my questions deeply, patiently, and with great understanding. He seemed to know so much more about the "big picture." After my friend had picked out the adoptive family, he seemed pleased that all was going as it should be.

He continually asked me to share with his biological family that he knew them all—mother, grandmother, father, uncle—and that he loved them dearly even though they may not see much of him after birth. He even knew the adoptive family by name. Love for all of them came flowing over me like ocean waves. They were the most intense feelings I think I have ever experienced. I couldn't help but break out in tears and shake all over. When I asked what he wanted me to call him, he told me "Kevin." Incidentally this is not the name chosen by the adoptive family. He said their name for him "was okay for out there, but for now you should call me Kevin."

I had never had much in the way of two-way conversations with the babies in my midwifery practice. They told me how to position the mother or warned me of complications. Except for the ones who announced their imminent delivery, and my subsequent begging to let me get my gloves on, there was no talking back from me to them. I guess I never even thought of talking back.

This baby was different. Most of the time when he talked to me I was just doing my usual chores when a feeling came over me and his words started spilling into my head, totally unsolicited and unexpected. Only a few times did he "zap me" while I was meditating.

I had never shared with anyone these experiences of talking with babies, but one day the grandmother was very upset and worried, crying about her daughter and the baby. I felt an overwhelming need to tell her, in little bits at first, in the hope that this would comfort her. And my hopes were realized. In fact, she shared this with Lynn and the grandfather and uncle. They all agreed that if they had heard of this from anyone else, they would have thought the person crazy, but since they have known me for so many years and knew of my clairvoyant abilities, this was indeed believable. In the end it was a matter of pure comfort for them all.

We even used a bit of humor—helpful in a situation like this! When they asked me how I received communication from the baby, the only way I could describe it was similar to "The Big Giant Head" on the TV show "Third Rock from the Sun." It just comes into my head and is so obviously this baby and not my imagination. So we joked about it, made the gestures for communicating with the Big Giant Head, but all knew it was a serious and true matter.

Much to their dismay, the baby would not tell me when he was coming. When I asked, he would reply, "I don't understand the question…. I will come when it is my time to come." I took this to mean that where he was, the concept of time is very different from ours. On two occasions when he came to me while I was meditating, I went with him to his "womb" instead of mine (pardon the pun). I could see the red/pink striations of the inside of the uterus through a milky veil (the amniotic bag). I could hear the maternal heartbeat and intestines. And, most amazing of all, I could clearly see Kevin's face! You can imagine my shock when he was delivered (actually when just his head was delivered) and he rotated his shoulders internally as babies do. I looked upon the very same face I had seen those two times in meditation. Now I know I shouldn't have been surprised, but I was about to fall over! I have to admit this in-utero conversation was a little too weird for me. I felt I had invaded the mother who had been invaded by the rapist months earlier, and I have not been able to tell her about that.

When the time for his birth came (an induction as the baby was overdue), the initiation of labor was slow. My friend asked me to go home for a while to check on my daughters. While there, I did a little meditation and sought out Kevin. This was the first time I initiated the conversation. I knew that no baby ever spoke to me after delivery of the head, so I wanted to say goodbye and also to ask how he was doing.

He kept telling me over and over, "I am afraid...I am afraid to come out. I think it will hurt and I know there will be a lot of sorrow from my mother when she gives me to the other family. I am afraid." I reassured him that the grandmother and I would be there with him and his mother the whole time and it was going to be all right. I told Kevin, "Yes, the parting will be painful, but the adoptive family loves you so very much. For all our pain, they have an equal measure of joy. Your birth will be okay. We will be there with you and your mama."

Only about thirty minutes after this conversation, my friend's mother called me to come back to hospital; labor had suddenly become intense and she wanted me. Kevin only talked to me once in labor, about a needed position change for Lynn because he was having trouble turning his head to get into the pelvis "this way." It was short and sweet, as so many other conversations with babies had been for me—specific in nature. After the position change, Lynn rapidly dilated from four centimeters to complete, and her four-and-a-half hour labor was soon over.

I miss Kevin very much and cannot help crying as I tell this story…

9

Working Things Out With Ezra

In the preceding chapters, we've taken an overview of pre-birth communication, from pre-conception through pregnancy to birth. Now we'll begin to look deeper, focusing on experiences that illuminate how we come together into families. Many of these stories involve a kind of dialogue between the unborn soul and the prospective parents—a process of coming to agreement. Sometimes the traces of this process are seen most clearly where there are problems, delays, and reversals.

The story of Miriam* and Steven is a good introduction to this dialogue. Working things out with their second child, Ezra, involved some serious negotiations before conception and further adjustments during the pregnancy. But to put Ezra's story in context, we must go back to relate the story of their first child, Asher, as told in *Soul Trek*. There we find a soul quietly, patiently courting a couple who have no intention of becoming parents.

Long before she married, Miriam realized she had a strong aversion to motherhood. She was so determined to avoid pregnancy that at the age of twenty-three she underwent tubal ligation. When she and Steven married, they agreed that children were not an option.

"For the first three years, we didn't give it another thought," says Steven. "It just felt right to be a couple." They worked with a series of counselors to improve their communication and mutual understanding. During individual sessions of Guided Imagery Through Music, their experiences were profound—and very different.

Miriam recalls: "My sessions seemed to center on past life memories. There were many horrible events surrounding pregnancy and childbirth, continual loss through dismal and violent means. After each session, the people acting as our guides had us draw a mandala or some other representation of the experience. My drawings were uniformly depressing.

"My final session was much different from all the others. A guide, obviously myself in fairy godmother garb, appeared and took me back to several of the figures I had identified with. She asked the people from the past to help me by keeping their fears, and sharing with me only their talents and positive aspects. It was incredibly healing, and it prepared me for my husband's relating his experience."

Steven picks up the story: "During one session, I saw a beautiful toddler with blond hair and blue eyes who held out an illuminated box containing a lotus flower. Afterwards, I drew a picture of this child. When I arrived home I showed Miriam the picture and told her that I had seen our baby. She was a bit taken aback, and suggested that a baby might be a metaphor for some new aspect in our lives. Besides, there hadn't been anyone with blue eyes in my family for three generations. I told her that I thought it was the image of a real baby.

"From then on, we both had numerous dreams and images of this child, and eventually decided to be open to his joining us." Steven and Miriam spent a year preparing for conception, reworking their health, environment, and relationship. Miriam underwent surgery to reverse the tubal ligation.

Says Steven, "We didn't 'hear' much from Asher during the time between his conception and his birth. As you might have guessed, he looked just like the picture I drew, blue eyes and all. Asher had his Barmitzvah earlier this month and has always been highly motivated about participating in this religious path. He's been an exceptional person since pre-conception and we cherish our relationship with him."

Courting Ezra—Miriam tells the story

Because Asher was so determined and patient in reaching us, we thought that was the way babies always announced themselves. Asher talked at an early age: individual words at ten months, sentences at one year. Before he was two, he told us that before he was born, he was "sitting with God" and said, "I want *them* to be my mama and my daddy." We had no reason to doubt him. So we waited.

About that same time, I went to see Ellie, a psychic whom a friend had recommended. I asked her if there was another child meant for us. She went into a light trance and vividly described a scene. She said that she saw a tenement around 1900. There were people everywhere, but she was looking at a little girl who was standing on the only spot of green, a tiny square of grass. From her description, the little girl resembled our son Asher. I explained to Ellie that I couldn't relate to this scene at all. My entire family, going back several generations, has been rural. No cities; certainly no tenements.

She said the little girl's name was Minnie. Immediate gooseflesh. My husband's family emigrated from Eastern Europe to Philadelphia. Everyone lived in the row houses of South Philly. Steven's grandmother was born in the early 1900's. Her name was Mae but everyone called her "Minnie." She had only one child, Steven's mother, and died when Steven was about fourteen. By all accounts she was a wonderful person, very smart, very determined.

After the session with Ellie, I was home doing laundry when Asher came into the laundry room. He said, "Mama, there's a baby girl living in our house. Do you ever see her?" Steven and I opened ourselves to pregnancy. We conceived three times, but each pregnancy ended within the first trimester.

About the time of the third loss, we got back in touch with an old friend, John Dye, naturopathic physician and midwife. He was a founder of the American Gentle Birthing Association and was sponsoring speakers and workshops in our hometown. We attended a lecture by Sondra Ray and decided to check out what John had to offer. John's program was very comprehensive. He had a co-management approach incorporating bodywork, rebirthing, talk therapy, guided imagery and birth education. (Those words seem so inadequate in describing the breadth of his program.) His goal was straightforward: No unwanted pregnancy—only conscious conception and an understanding of the context of each birth.

One thing that came up for me as soon as we started working together was the reality of Asher's birth. The conception and pregnancy had been wonderful, but the labor was a thirty-eight hour ordeal of excruciating low back pain. I remembered that I had vowed never to go through that again. John assured me that I need not. He told me that acupuncture could solve that problem and he would be there for me if I needed that intervention. That alone lifted a huge burden.

Together, Steven and I did a few sessions of guided imagery with John. We asked for contact if there was a baby meant to join us. We asked what was needed to induce this being to accept physical form. We received such amazingly similar answers! At the end of one session, we sat up and looked at each other incredulously. "A four-door car?" we said in unison. This child had many safety issues, one of which was the need to replace our two-door car with one with four doors.

We also heard very clearly that this child didn't trust us. "You promised my brother many things such as a home in the country, but you still live in the city." We immediately started making plans to move to a rural area. We put our house on the market and took a loss in order to be able to move as soon after the birth as we could (we didn't want to move before the birth since we wanted John in attendance).

It was after the house was on the market that we got pregnant. Because of the previous miscarriages, we waited until we were in our second trimester to tell Asher.

"Oh, I know. His name is Ezra Aaron."

"What if we have a girl?"

"His name is Ezra Aaron," Asher nodded, smiling.

"Do you know anyone named Ezra?"

"No. That's just his name."

Asher was the only one who seemed to think it was a boy. People were stopping me on the street, telling me that I was going to have a girl.

Asher had a game he played with the baby. He'd put his little hand on my belly and say, "Hey baby! This is your big brother. Give me a whap!" And wherever he had his hand, the baby would kick or punch him. They seemed to be having a great time together right from the start.

A midwife who was on the birth team came to interview Steven and me, both individually and together. We explored concepts such as what does it mean to be a "mother," "father," "parent." Our interviews totaled a few hours of exploring stereotypes and refining goals and values. We were also assigned to talk with our own parents. We had specific questions assigned, such as "What was the family situation around the time of my conception?" "What do you remember about my conception?" "What do you remember about my birth?" "Did you plan my conception?" We learned both from the answers and from the resistance that some parents showed to the questions.

We had never had a sonogram with Asher, but we did with our second baby. John did one in his office, but the image wasn't clear enough for him so he referred me to a hospital for imaging. Looking back, I regret having done it, but that's just another "oh well" in the personal history. We got a very clear picture of the swimmer. The tech asked if we wanted to know if it was a boy or girl, but it was so obvious, she didn't need to say. Ezra Aaron indeed!

That night I felt the baby go breech. The next morning I called John. He had me come in for an external version. Once he got me on the slant board, he and his partner, Ed Hofmann-Smith, started talking to us about why a baby would go breech. They said that in their many years of experience they had noted that babies go breech when they are the sex other than what their parents wanted. As if to say, "Here! Note this and see if you can accept me."[1] We protested immediately that we had not *wanted* a girl; there was no attachment on our part to either sex. "Tell him," they both advised.

So while they listened to the baby's heartbeat with the Doppler and guided the little swimmer, both Steven and I told him that we loved him for who he is. I turned to Steven and said, "As long as he's healthy, I don't care." John said, "What if he's *not* healthy?" Hmmmm. That took a moment of sorting. "That doesn't matter either. As long as he's who he is." "Tell him." So we talked on until the procedure was completed.

"Well," said Ed, "we'll see if he believes you." Apparently the baby would go breech if he didn't believe us. That evening, while meditating, I realized that Ezra was the one who was having a hard time with the news. I think he hadn't read the fine print: that this time around he was a boy. Steven and I determined that we would reinforce as often as possible that we are happy with him as he is—that there is nothing about him we want to change.

When Ezra was born, Asher and Steven cut the cord. Ez was alert and curious from the start. He stayed awake for a couple of hours while the whole crew oohed and ahhed over his beauty. He made eye contact with each of them. After the hubbub died away and everyone had packed up and left, Asher climbed up on the bed where I was sitting holding Ezra. He gently stroked the baby's head and said, "God made us brothers so we can be friends forever."

Since then, Steven and I have often thought that these boys are here for each other. We are privileged to be witnesses of their processes. As I write this, I am listening to the radio program Performance Today. A beautiful arrangement of "Appalachian Spring" is playing. It has a recurring theme of the Quaker song, "Tis the Gift to be Simple." I am filled with the understanding that it is important for me to retell this story for my own benefit as well as for Ezra's. Each of us, as John Dye stressed, deserves to be wanted. Thank you for the opportunity.

10

The Dialogue of Agreement

Pre-birth communication stories are full of clues about the processes that bring an unborn soul into a specific family. However, the clues don't all point to one overarching picture. If you love a good mystery, you'll enjoy exploring them with me, but you won't find pat answers here.

Do we (for example) really choose each other? It would be splendid to announce that all the evidence shows us choosing our parents and selecting the circumstances of our lives, yet this isn't so. Contradictions abound. If we gather soul memory stories, and add reports from people experiencing hypnotic regression, the answer is both yes and no. Alongside memories of choosing and memories of being guided by a wise counselor, there are accounts in which the pairing seems unconscious or even random.

My best guess is that there is some measure of choice, but maybe not in every case. Perhaps the Tibetan lama has it right who explains: "The choice of parents is not always a voluntary one. Yet in the intermediate state, imprints and karma ripen and attract us. When there is clarity of mind in life and death, then there is clarity in choice of parents."[1]

That said, there remains plenty of evidence that choosing, accommodating, and negotiating do go on between potential parents and unborn souls as they prepare to become a family. You will find this evidence in the stories to come. You'll read of experiences that suggest what I believe to be true: that there is much freedom, flexibility, and creativity in our soul's existence, and that in varying degrees we do choose or at least participate in planning our lives.

What logic brings us together? One possibility, of course, is that a greater intelligence assigns us to families, for reasons beyond our limited view. The coming of a child is sometimes announced by such a wise presence rather than by the unborn soul itself. In childhood, Francine was directed by an inner voice to remember her pre-existence. That same voice, which Francine thinks of as the voice of her heavenly mother, has continued to guide and console her at critical times. She writes:

> I had two children, a son and a daughter. Paul was severely autistic and I thought I had my hands full and didn't have room in my life for another child. Wrong! The "voice" worked on me for almost a year with a simple message that repeated every night and throughout the days: "A child is waiting." It's a long story, but the end of it is that we had our third child, Robert, who has been a tremendous blessing and has given us strength and purpose, especially after the death of our first son, Paul.

Like Francine, a reluctant parent who yields to such persistence may discover unexpected gifts. This was the case for Israeli journalist Noa Bareket. After her two sons were born, she felt that she didn't want any more children, but then, four years later…

Noa: An old and wise soul

> I was talking with a friend when suddenly she looked at me and said that she saw this beautiful girl who was about to be my daughter. I was amazed and told her I wasn't planning to have more kids, but she was sure, and for a second I could imagine that girl.
>
> I started dreaming about her. She wanted to come and I would say no, I can't, don't have the money, time, energy, and space for you—but she insisted. Finally after almost a year I told a friend

about this. My friend asked if I wanted to have her and I replied that I was afraid. She asked, "If you believe children choose their parents, can you not trust this soul to know what is right for her?" I do believe our children choose us. My friend went on, "She knows you don't have much money and you live in a small house and you have a career that you love, and if she wants to come - why not?" I felt relief, and a couple of weeks later I took out the IUD. I soon became pregnant.

A few days after making love, as I was walking, suddenly the light became bright and I felt her. She was happy and thanked me for being her mother. I felt that she was a very old and wise soul and that she is more advanced than I am. A couple of weeks later, while I was taking a shower, suddenly the light changed again and the name Miriam came to my mind. I never loved this name and knew only old ladies with it, but she told me that this is her name. I kept this to myself because I thought my husband would laugh at me. A month passed and one morning he said, "I have this crazy name for her"—it was Miriam!

She is now three and a half years old, and her name is hers, no doubt about it. She brought happiness and prosperity with her to my family and I thank God for her.

Some stories have "destiny" written all over them, such as this account from *Parenting Begins Before Conception* by Carista Luminare:

One night I was lying in bed waiting for my husband to come home. I felt a presence at the foot of the bed, while simultaneously a warm light flooded my whole body. My heart expanded with a feeling of compassion for an image of a small baby who smiled at me. We had a silent understanding that we would be parent and child, and then a series of insights was unleashed about who this being was, when she wanted to be conceived, and what she wanted to be named. But most alarming was that she imparted to me an undeniable sense that my husband, Jerry, was not the father, and that it would be two and a half years before the conditions would be aligned for her arrival into my life...Sure enough, almost two and a half years to the day later, Sasha was born into the arms of her father, my new husband of three months.

An experience like this certainly implies that our children are pre-destined to join us; yet even these arrangements may not be set in stone. Many stories suggest a give and take, a mutual choosing with freedom on both sides. I think of it as a dialogue between ourselves and the souls wishing to be born. Much of this dialogue may take place outside of our conscious awareness, but some of it appears to us as an experience of pre-birth communication.

While some communications seem to come from children who are determined to join a specific family, others show souls finding alterna-tive paths if their first choice is blocked. I like to emphasize this free-dom, because occasionally I hear from someone who is disturbed by sensing the presence of a potential child. Carmen* was feeling a little frantic when she wrote:

> I feel all alone about this. I am thirty-five years old, and I strongly believed that I would never want children at all. I have recently met a man who definitely wants children, and he thinks I am ready for them. I don't know if it's my age and the biological clock, or the fact that I have never before been with a man who wanted children, who made me feel secure and who seems like he would be an amaz-ing father...But I have begun to have this feeling of a presence or spirit hanging over my shoulder, being with me, watching me. I don't know if this man is the father, but I am obviously the mother. I suddenly feel alone, like I need this other being, this part of me.
>
> Please tell me what is happening. I feel like my body and my hormones have taken over my mind. I can't stop thinking about babies and children. It's actually driving me a little crazy. Are there other women I can talk to about this? Are there books? Websites? Is this normal? And can I trust these new feelings, after a lifetime of being committed to being childless? Please help...

My response to Carmen sums up my thoughts on freedom of choice for all souls (born and unborn) who are considering conception: "First of all, I would say...relax. You will be able to sense what's right for you much better if you can take it easy and quiet your mind. You may be experiencing the presence of a soul wishing to join you; what you describe is typical of this. But there is no need to feel pressured or that you must make an instant decision. Relax, tune in to the presence you feel, have a conversation with it and express your doubts and questions. Your desires and the child's intentions are both important. If it isn't right for you to have a child, there are other options for a soul wanting to be born."

Tara's story illustrates the spaciousness and generosity that exist within the adventure of coming to birth. It also introduces a pattern we will explore in later chapters—the connection between unborn souls and grandparents in spirit.

Tara* S: A place filled with light

When I met my partner and soulmate I knew we would have two children: a little girl and a little boy. We hadn't really planned on getting pregnant right away.

I was lying in bed one night meditating and a small voice in my right ear said, "My name is Emily." I thought initially she was a ghost. I said hello in my mind (Roy* was sound asleep next to me and I didn't want to wake him or have him think I'd gone off the deep end) and asked what she was here for.

She said, "You're going to have a daughter." I said, "Really? I would love to have a daughter. Who will be the father?" She giggled and said, "With Roy, silly." I smiled, and just felt bathed in love and light. I woke Roy and told him I'd dreamed we would have a daughter. He sleepily reminded me that he couldn't have children (he had tried in a previous marriage). I told him again that we would have a daughter. He said he hoped so and went back to sleep.

And really, since that moment, she has been with me all the time. A full year and a half later we found out we were pregnant. Quite by accident, let me assure you; I was on the pill and Roy had been told he was not able to have children. We were shocked. It shook me to the core and I can only imagine what it did for Roy.

We still had a lot going on in both of our lives: he was finishing up a divorce and taking care of his three children that he had with his first wife (they used donor insemination); I was in the process of building a career, and it just seemed overwhelming. We weren't sure what to do and it became such that the thought of keeping her was harder than the thought of giving her back to God.

I cried and cried and cried and the worst part of it was that I couldn't hear Emily any more. I went to church and sat in the back pew and prayed to God. I told Him how sorry I was, that I didn't want to give Emily back, but I just wasn't sure I could make it. I wasn't sure Roy and I would make it, that we had any chance of being a family.

I heard a sigh and then, "I never stop loving my children, no matter what their choices are." And at that moment I had a strong vision of being in a place filled with soft, white light and I saw my grandfather, as I remember him from childhood, holding the hand of a little girl of about five years old. She had long blond hair (both Roy and I are blond) and blue, blue eyes. I knew she was mine. I also knew that God would take care of her until I was ready to. I knew she would be safe with my grandfather and that he would watch over her. I was filled with a sense of peace about it all.

After much soul-searching we decided to have the baby. I'm only thirteen weeks along and my friends ask me how I know it's a girl, how I got the vision. I tell them I've always had visions and I see things differently than most people. I tell them it's like listening to music. You hear a song once and you simply know you like it, or you know you don't. I assure them that if they will quiet their own thoughts and concentrate, they will find they know things, too. It just takes practice.

As for keeping the lines of communication open, I do still meditate. Nothing too fancy, but I quiet myself and regulate my breathing and just relax into where I'm at—into myself, I suppose. I always have questions to ask and when I find that my thoughts about the day or tomorrow have died down, I ask them. The trick is not to discount what you hear when they are answered.

Emily talks to me every now and then. When I told her we would like to call her Elizabeth instead because Roy doesn't like the name Emily, she said that was all right, but could we please spell it with an 's' instead of a 'z'? No problem, I assured her. She tells me she is doing well and she is growing. I know she will be an amazing person, one of those people in life who hold others together and make sense out of things that others can't understand. I am proud she has chosen my partner and me to be her parents, and I can't wait to see her little face.

Emily/Elisabeth was born in the spring of 2001, a healthy girl just as promised.

11

Yes, No, Maybe So

Many pre-conception contacts are gentle and unassuming requests to join the family. They offer us a chance to welcome the child, postpone conception for a while, or firmly close the door. The following stories illustrate these varying responses to an unborn soul applying for admission.

Karen: Tiny Kisses

A couple of months ago I was taking a nap and having an explicit sex dream about myself and my husband, similar to the ones I had before I got pregnant with my son. While I was observing this dream I felt tiny kisses on my hands. These were the same kinds of kisses that I, and about nine other people, had felt at a spiritual retreat this past spring.

I immediately woke up and shouted out loud, "Oh no! You're not going to talk me into having another baby. I'm too old and too tired!" The kisses continued and I tried to brush them away. This time I spoke silently in my head. "NO! I know there are special babies waiting to be born but I cannot have any more babies at this time. But I do have a friend…If she gives her permission you can go see her." The kisses stopped—and so have those dreams.

I told the friend about the dream. She laughed, hopefully didn't think I was totally crazy, and said she would have to talk to her husband. I pray there are women out there, ones younger and less tired than I am, who are willing and ready to accept these remarkable souls who are yearning to come to earth. Those women must be able to accept that these children, like my five-year-old son, know what they want ("to protect the world from the bad guys") and who they are ("When I grow up, I'm going to be a ninja, a storyteller and a great singer"), and be prepared to nurture their extraordinary talents ("I just talked to the healing angels and they're going to go help our Grandma who is sick").

Beatrice*: A graceful no thank you

When my son was one and a half years old, I was with my family where a lady was present who did readings. (My son was not there; he was at home with his aunt.) I asked for a reading but did not tell her what I was wondering—did I make the right choice in keeping my child after birth, as I was a young mother.

So I sat with her as she told me I was to have two children in my life, one a boy, the other a girl. The boy would come first, and the girl later. They would be far apart with two different fathers. I was impressed with her unknowing "hit" as far as my son was concerned, but was skeptical about ever having a second child, as I knew I would need to dedicate most of my life to the early arrival of my son and all the "catching up" I'd have to do to stabilize myself financially after taking on the responsibilities of motherhood at an early age.

Six years later, I was remarried to my present husband/soulmate, and it was after seven years of marriage that my pre-birth communication occurred. I awoke suddenly from a wonderful, touching dream where a little baby girl came to me and asked if I would like to be her mother, as she had picked a few sets of possible parents. She appeared as a young image of about one or two years old. She had pale ash blond hair and hazel eyes and she was very beautiful, inwardly and outwardly. She seemed to be covered in an almost translucent, shimmery gossamer-like material, like a small gown. I felt the soul resonance of her personality and how curious she was about relationships between souls, and sensed she was mainly going to be a student of humanities in some form.

I was deeply touched by her request and a part of me liked the idea of a little girl, but I felt I could not give her all that she might need. I felt sad that I was not in a position to enjoy having her in our lives, and told her if there were any way I could, I would love to welcome her and love her. She was very loving towards me and understood my reasons, and let me know she would be "okay" as she had a set of parents chosen as backup.

She floated softly away in my dream as I sent her my love and I woke up in awe of such an experience with such a wonderful soul. I told my husband about her and he agreed it would have been lovely to have her, our own little girl, but we both felt we were not in a position to give her the best. We were still relatively young parents, striving to accomplish some goals in our careers. We were dedicating a lot of time to assure my son's success at overcoming his learning differences, and making sure he was happy and got lots of attention. So we knew we just couldn't give her the time she would also deserve.

I was honored she approached me in the way she did, and I know she is now alive and well on earth. I am not aware of where she has taken birth, but I was at home one afternoon when, in the middle of doing something, I got a flash through me like the "astral post" of her having safely and happily arrived into life that day. She was letting me know she'd made it and was here, as if saying, "Don't worry, I'm all right."

The dialogue of agreement can be simple and swift. Shawna Stewart and her husband had always wanted five children. After reaching number five, they began to use birth control. But one night after making love, Shawna had "a wondrous experience: I heard a voice of a little boy asking me if I would be his mother. I felt this was a soul reaching out to me. I said, quietly, 'I'd love to' and that's when my little boy Caden and I first met." Caden was conceived that night and Shawna says, "He has been a blessing for the whole family, gentle and loving."

When a soul reaches out in this way, we have the option of welcoming it into our lives but asking it to wait a while. We can postpone conception while staying in touch with the unborn soul. This was the experience of Rob and Jill, whose story was first introduced in Chapter One.

Rob and Jill: "If we make love right now…"

A few months ago, my fiancé and I were lying in bed and simply relaxing. We began kissing and were both inspired to move on to bigger and better activities. All of a sudden, I had the most beautiful, warm, and tingly feeling. I knew I had felt a child, our child, in the room with us. I immediately stopped Rob and said, "If we make love right now, we are going to have a baby." I was surprised when he said, "I know."

Rob and I both felt nothing extraordinary in a physical sense, maybe just a warmth or, for me, a ticklish feeling in my uterus. It was more an emotional/spiritual experience for us. The cool thing is that, although it was amazing, it wasn't a foreign feeling at all. In fact, we agreed the feeling was familiar and totally unique at the same time. It was literally like a wash of a loving, powerful, and familiar presence over us. From what we can determine, we felt very similar things and at the same time.

At that moment, we chose to wait. Since then, we have talked about that spirit who visited us. We both agreed that it was a girl. I have had contact with her since then, through images in my mind's eye. We plan to get married and move to Hawaii within the next year and then begin our family.

The most recent contact she has made with me was to tell me her name. Rob and I were confident she would make her name known to us and she did! I wasn't really thinking about names and then her name just popped into my head and I knew. I said it out loud: "Laurel…" It sounded so right. I told Rob that she had given me her name and he asked what it was. I was too afraid to speak it to him—what if he didn't like the name she had already chosen?! So I spelled it for him and he said it and a huge smile came over his face. He knew it was perfect…Laurel Evelyn Butterworth.

Rob and I have discussed the reasons we are blessed with these "meetings." We think it is simply because we are open to them and we live in a space of love, at least some of the time. We know we are the conscious creators of our lives and that a child will be consciously welcomed into our lives in perfect timing. We respect our child spirit as a powerful being and we respect her choice to be with us. She will be an equal partner in our decision to have her join us in this realm.

About two years later, Jill announced, "I am happy to say that Laurel Evelyn has indeed joined us and is now almost seven months old. She is exactly as she told us she would be and just how I saw her in my mind and dreams."

We have many ways of responding to a soul's advances, and our potential children have a charming variety of ways to approach us. The first time an unborn soul introduced itself to Elana Sabajon, it announced its intention to join her in such a matter-of-fact way that Elana hardly felt she was given a choice! A few years later, a second child approached in a very different manner that made it comfortable for Elana and Ravi to request a postponement. Here, she tells the story of both these meetings.

Elana: Dancing in the valley

It was in October 1997 that I participated at a meditation workshop, two to three hours per evening on four consecutive days. Each night I had a vision.

In my first vision, I was on a path surrounded by light, flowers, trees, sunshine, butterflies and a crowd of children. I did not make too much of it, because at the time I was working in my own classroom as a Montessori directress. In my second vision, a soul came up to me in the void and introduced itself (notice there was no gender!), telling me that it chose my partner Ravi and myself to be its parents, and that s/he would like to arrive soon. The third day she told me she was going to be a girl and the fourth day she also told me her name: Gloria.

I had my period a week earlier than usual on those four days and it was the best flow I ever had, cleansing and freeing, just great! I felt spiritually and mentally pregnant. My partner and I did not necessarily plan to have children at the time. I had just started work towards my Master's degree. Anyhow, I felt the exact time I ovulated, we conceived, a girl was born and her name is Gloria.

Early this spring I had another experience. Energy surrounded me. Again I felt it was a soul energy, introducing itself as wanting to be born as a male child. I also had a dream about the name, which was rather an unusual name, somewhat like Armentis, or Armantes. Not only did I feel the excitement of a spiritual pregnancy in me—this time I felt completely overwhelmed and a fear of not being able to follow this call right now in my life. I am trying to cope with finishing my MA and looking after Gloria, and a pregnancy on top of this just does not seem manageable to me. I felt torn inside.

My first experience with Gloria's soul is sacred and special to me. I feel humbled that I was able and allowed to have such a sacred interaction with Gloria's soul. And then this. I felt that if I denied this soul's request, I would deny the Divine to enter.

I talked to my partner about it. Strangely enough, he had started speaking about a second child during this time frame as well. We talked it over and decided I would try to contact the soul. I spoke to the soul, letting him know that I was honored and asked him if he could wait another three months or so, as that would help me greatly. Since that encounter I do not feel spiritually pregnant. I even felt a little bit sad to let go. I hoped this soul was not "turned off," and would either choose another set of parents or return to us later in life.

The difference between my first experience with Gloria's soul and the second experience was that it was not in a setting of visions. It was rather energy that I felt, thoughts and little visions in meditations or during everyday life, and a dream with the name. Gloria's soul was hardly giving me a choice, while this time it seemed to me more as if the soul was knocking at the door, expressing a wish and hoping.

A need arose in me to contact the soul once more and to make sure everything was all right. I was meditating and putting out the request to connect again with this particular spirit. I had a beautiful vision of a woman with long dark hair, floating white skirt, looking somewhat like me, dancing in this beautiful valley (which I always call *my* valley, with grass, flowers, mountains, water, and animals).

However, you could hardly see the surroundings because she was dancing amongst all these soul energies waiting to be born. I got a deep, deep feeling of unconditional love sent to me, as if saying: "I am fine, I am waiting." I felt very blessed and at ease.

In a second vision this woman and I were dancing alone in the middle of something, which at first I could not recognize. We were dancing somewhat self-absorbed. I began to feel lonely and sad, when I realized that we had an audience. Female and male Masters, Jesus among them, and a very old man whom I could not identify and lots of women, also undefined, were standing around us, watching us, moving to the music, smiling lovingly, when a male voice very clearly told me: "You are taken care of, do not worry, you are not alone."

Elana announced her pregnancy later in the year, and her new daughter was born the following June.

One of the joys of pre-birth communication is the sense of meeting a personality as mature and understanding as oneself (or considerably more so!), whose perspective comes from beyond the limits of a body. Sometimes we think there's no place in our life for a child, but the contact itself brings such sweetness that it changes us, opens the heart and makes us ready. A Canadian woman describes her experience:

Paula: "When are you going to be ready for me?"

My son Timothy is now just a little over two years of age. I feel as though I have known him for much longer. About two years before his conception, I was in the exciting beginning of my career as a psychotherapist. Enjoying my "calling" and growing through my own issues of being adopted, I decided I did not want to have any children.

One night I had a very vivid dream. A toddler (who looked remarkably like my son does now) appeared to me and said, "Mommy, when are you going to be ready for me?"

I replied, "Who are you?"

"I am Timothy, your son."

I awoke startled…startled and almost instantaneously differ-ent—changed. I felt a beautiful sense of peace and of love.

He appeared in my dreams often until I conceived (without planning) about a year later. Now I have started to mobilize myself to re-enter the outside work force, as I am a full-time mother at home. However, I am halted with what appears to be dreams of a little girl letting me know she will be with me soon. Again I have a warm, peaceful, loving, transformational feeling. It is also very humbling, as I feel like a small part of a very large, magnificent whole.

I thought I was the only one. I have always had intuitive experi-ences; they are really the cornerstones of my existence. Motherhood is indeed spiritual for me and I am eternally grateful. Incidentally, I have endometriosis and my doctors find it quite remarkable that I conceived. I don't. I knew Timothy was to come.

12

Courting the Couple: Sarah and Liam's Story

There is a kind of pre-birth communication that I like to call the court-ing dance, where contacts continue over an extended period of time until at last the child is conceived. In such cases it's quite common for the pregnancy to be "quieter" than pre-conception, almost as though the soul can relax and breathe a sigh of contentment once that's settled.

Sarah* and Liam* are a young couple living in the Southwest of the United States. Sarah is a writer and a graduate student in Transper-sonal Psychology; Liam an eclectic writer, banker, and retired breeder of thoroughbred horses. Our correspondence began in January, 2000, when Sarah introduced herself and explained her dilemma: although she was not at all sure she wanted to be a mother, there seemed to be a soul courting her with patient persistence. The story unfolds over time and is especially interesting because both Sarah and Liam felt the soul's advances. Sarah began:

> For the past three years I've sensed the presence of a being who wishes for us to be its parents. Although I am a nurturing person by nature, I've not really wanted to parent a child in this life, probably the result of feeling as if I parented my mother. Regardless, I sense there is a contractual agreement with this being. I've dreamed about this soul and I've had intuitive moments where I seem to be receiving its energy more openly. But I am hesitant to parent, not

because I feel I would be a bad parent, but because I realize the level of responsibility that such a task entails.

I wonder about the nature of free will in this sort of circumstance. In the case of a spiritual agreement such as this appears to be, is there an option for free will to play a part at all? And I wonder if it is my ego resisting, or perhaps some other aspect of myself. There are moments when I do feel receptive, but then, they are just moments.

Dear Sarah (I replied), from what I've learned, there seems to be an active process of agreement between souls and potential parents. Are these agreements rigid and binding? I do not think they are. I sometimes hear from women who sense the presence of a soul and feel obligated to bear a child they really do not want. I point them to evidence that other doorways may be available for those who need to be born.

Your dilemma is also about whether you want to have a child. Like you, I had an inner struggle around the issue of whether or not I wanted to be a mother. I doubted my ability to do a good job of it, and I wasn't particularly fond of babies and children. For me, having children was a revelation. Before, I thought mostly of what parenthood would involve in terms of giving and giving up. Afterwards, I found out it's a two-way street, a mutual exchange.

Dear Elisabeth (Sarah wrote), reminding me that the exchange between parent and child is mutual, helped me today in opening my heart to the possibility of parenting. It was a significant shift for me, and I am grateful.

As for the details of my "soul contact" experience, I'd like to give you some background first. My own psychic and intuitive experiences began when I was very young; at ages four and five are my earliest memories of the beings on the other side of what I perceived as a veil. I have had a sort of fluid exposure between the various levels of spiritual worlds that exist, though I don't pretend to understand the levels and dimensions well.

My dream life has always been vivid and fulfilling, and during my early teens I began to work at uncovering the deeper meanings of my dreams. I discovered there were several levels of dreaming for me, and I began to decipher the differences between psychic dreams and other levels. Up until a few years ago, I always interpreted my "child" dreams as archetypal, as if it were my own inner child relating messages to me. Then something clicked and I realized that in certain dreams there was a soul contacting me.

The energy of the child has been intense and purposeful. Usually I see it as male, but on two occasions the soul has appeared as female. The dreams are lucid; I have some degree of control over the events and conversation. Communication in the dreams is telepathic rather than verbal.

The dreams have been on and off for three years, yet they are not the times when I feel the being most strongly. Those times are usually mundane moments—washing dishes, sweeping the floor and so on. It's just a sense that something is there; it is a child-like energy, not my own, and it is hovering close.

At one point, there was a nightly occurrence that was quite curious and I know this soul was the cause of it. Right after we'd settle down for bed I would hear a bang and clash in the back bedroom (the room my partner and I designated as the "maybe-future-baby" room). In college I had made a carved ceramic tile of a pregnant woman with beautifully wild hair, sitting on a bed of grapes with the vines twining through her locks. She's in her ninth month. Well, the tile made its falling-off-the-secure-post performance regularly for several nights in a row, without ever cracking!

Finally, I told the soul I wasn't ready, that I was working on my own growth and in doing so, perhaps I would come to a revelation that I did want to parent. I felt that the being understood, and there were no more tile events. I also heard in my mind that there was a time frame offered, a window. I haven't sensed the being around recently, and have wondered if the time frame has passed. Part of me doesn't think so, for when I wonder about it, I've had a sort of waking dream about being pregnant. In this waking dream, I am thirty-one years old, and that's about two years away. Also, I'm not living in my present location and the people around me are not people I know right now.

My partner, Liam, has dreamed about this soul as well, and curiously enough, up until the past three years he has not wanted to have children. Liam is very intuitive and sensed this soul's energy for a few months before mentioning it to me. We laughed when we realized we had been sensing the same energy! He has dreamed of the being as a boy, and once as a girl. We both have felt that this soul has a very determined sense of mission. Liam has told me he is now open to the idea of being a parent.

We've both felt our being's energy as quite intense. We've also felt a playfulness along with the intensity, but usually there is a sense of pointed awareness. In my night dreams, the being is often a young boy of about two or three with dark hair and green eyes, and he has a very solemn look to him as if he drinks in the world through his eyes and holds all of its events and memories within them. He is usually quite calm and still. He has love in his eyes too, and in a few dreams I've seen sadness as well.

In waking life when I sense the being's presence, it is similar to the feeling of someone standing behind you while you're doing something and you suddenly feel you aren't alone in the room and turn to look. It's that point of recognition, that moment, I feel the most, except the moment is suspended through a longer period of time.

I've often wondered if I will experience the "ready" feeling that others seem to express. There are days when I feel I might be close, but then something shifts in me and I seem to move away from feeling ready into feeling so not ready. I've met so many women who've had difficulty in their relationships with their mothers, and difficulty parenting as a result, and I've wondered if part of being ready for me has to do with trusting that I've grown through therapy in the past ten years, so I will not mother like my own mother.

Oh yes, the fear of repeating those old patterns! I confess I'm a dreadful mother in many ways. I've made many mistakes. My children have been burdened and distorted by my own fears and my lack of patience. Sometimes I half-jokingly remind my daughter that she chose me, after all. (She hotly denies it!) But the concept that our children may have chosen us is comforting, when we worry that other parents would be better for them.

If we suppose that our children are souls coming with their own intentions, it gives a different feeling to the parent role. With my daughter, for example, from about the second day after her birth I began to feel she was somehow older than I am. She seems to know about the world and to be comfortable with life in a way that's beyond me. The idea that my children existed before they came to me subtly changes how I relate to them. It softens that feeling of awesome responsibility that can be so intimidating.

> May 2000…This soul who is petitioning for us to be its parents is getting very active. The being came to Liam a couple of nights ago in a dream and said this: "I am an intelligent soul and I don't want any baby talk when I get there please. I've been around the block a few times and would appreciate being talked to in an intelligent manner."

> September…The baby will be coming sooner rather than later. It has told me that it needs to be here by the end of next year and would prefer to be a Sagittarius if at all possible!

By October Sarah and Liam move to a new house in a new town. (Remember her image of being in a different place when pregnant?) Mid-October Sarah writes:

> Not too much news on the soul contact front. I do feel that the babe will be here by the end of next year though. Probably my biggest sense of sadness comes from not having a relationship with strong female figures in my life to accompany me through this woman's passage. My mother and I don't have a relationship and Liam doesn't have a relationship with his mother. Even if we did, I don't feel they would be particularly loving or supportive. Though I know I will have Liam, a part of me yearns for a female community too as I take this step.
>
> In the meantime, the bathtub has been stripped and refinished, we've repainted just about everything in joyful colors and we're adding another bathroom/laundry room and a new kitchen. My hands are full!
>
> Tell me what you love about motherhood and what you don't love about it in your next letter. I'm curious to hear.

Yesterday was my birthday and having my son here for several days made it special. He is nearly twenty-one and my daughter is fourteen. They are so loving and really like good friends. This is the best part: I feel nourished by the love I feel for them. The parts that have been hard: knowing I've made mistakes and harmed them in various ways. There's no way to undo the damage I have caused by being an imperfect mother!

The early years with each one, when children need almost total attention, it was sometimes difficult for me to deal with the demands, especially when I was trying to do something involving thinking or creativity. A certain amount of frustration and isolation comes into it then. Not being able to count on time alone was hard for me, but definitely worth it. They are the light of my life.

November 13…Last night, I dreamed I had a baby girl. The baby told me it was thinking of trying out the female gender because it seemed it would be more fun to be a female. The baby was six pounds, two ounces. It's been neat having communication with this soul. I am feeling it won't be too long now before it takes its human form.

November 29…A good friend of Liam's phoned last night to ask if I was pregnant! He said he dreamed I was pregnant with a baby girl and she told him she would be a Virgo. Funny, because I said to Liam that I think a Virgo would be very good for both of us, personality-wise (not that I know a thing about Virgos!). We've not discussed having a child with those around us, so his friend had no idea we were even thinking about it.

December 26…I have good news…I'm going to be a mother! I just found out last week and am thrilled. Looks like this soul really, really wanted to be here as we only tried once. I've been very calm and am wondering if this calmness is part of the personality of this child.

January 2001…I'm about seven weeks along and feeling very calm and happy about it. All is going well with the pregnancy and

I've had no morning sickness at all and have been able to continue my usual six mile canyon walks twice a week, though I've had to back off on the ashtanga yoga because of the increased tiredness. Liam and I are going for our first appointment with the midwife next week and we've already checked out the birthing center, which looks like a B&B and has a water birthing tub available. The interesting thing about it is that up until the time I became pregnant I seemed to have more contact with the soul who wants to be the babe. Now, I've had none that I can recall.

February…I'm in my thirteenth week of pregnancy and we just heard the baby's heartbeat the other day—Liam was moved to tears—it was very dear. I'm still feeling great. We took a water birth class last week and I'm feeling really good about it for my process. We're still debating about whether or not we want a doula at the birth. Still no contact from the soul itself, though a good friend of mine says it has contacted her and she feels very connected to this soul.

June…I asked the soul that is our child what it wanted to be named and it gave me the most atrocious names in a dream: Alouicious if a boy, and Ezmerelda May if a girl. And then it giggled in such a delightful childish way when I paused in the dream feeling like "NO WAY!" When I asked, "Are you serious?!" the soul said in a light but clearly adult voice this time, "Name me what you want, I'll be happy with whatever name you choose. It will just be fun to be together."

September—Dear Sarah, I'm excited that the birth is so near. I hope you will have lots of very private time with just Liam and baby and you, afterwards. I hope you know some people who will bring over a lovely meal, say, "Ooh, pretty baby" and then leave. Or, if not, make some cheese blintzes and freeze them this week! I have an indelible memory of breakfast in bed that Nick would bring me: cheese blintzes with sour cream and cherries and a cup of chai…Pure heaven, with baby alongside. Heaven should be like that.

Liam and I have prepared some frozen delights and have let everyone (including all family members) know that we are taking two
weeks in seclusion to bond with our new sweetie. Most people
seemed very surprised, but those who know us well know this is a
very special time for us and they honor and respect our choice.
Liam has taken two months of paternity leave (which shocked his
boss and co-workers) so we'll have a lovely two months!

Liam and Sarah's daughter was born at the beginning of September
(remember their friend who dreamed that the baby told him she would
be a girl born in Virgo!). Sarah's labor was long and hard but at the end
of it, "they placed her directly on me as soon as she came out and her
eyes were wide open and she just looked at me. I just cried—it is the
most amazing and magnificent thing I have ever experienced in my life.
I am in awe of the beauty of this and it feels as if my heart has opened
in a way that I cannot explain. Wow, life is beautiful and nothing will
ever be the same or look the same or feel the same again."

13

Miscarriage

Miscarriage is such a common event, the fate of at least one in six pregnancies—common enough to be a normal chapter in a woman's childbearing years. Yet I was unprepared when it happened to me, as though I'd never known this was a possible outcome. Irrationally, I felt like I was the only person who had ever miscarried, and there seemed to be no support or information available.

A friend briskly advised me to get right back into my normal life. Though it was kindly meant, I felt misunderstood and more alone. I needed to hear that it was not self-indulgent but good to rest and comfort myself and grieve. At my medical check, even the doctor and nurse lacked empathy. They seemed puzzled and disapproving when I burst into tears as the last remnants of my long-desired pregnancy were reamed out.

This kind of emotional isolation makes losing a pregnancy more painful than it has to be. The personal experiences of miscarriage need acknowledgment, and I am glad that in recent years they have come out of the shadows to be spoken more freely.

The Soul's Decision?

We think of miscarriage as a failure, a failed pregnancy. Could it sometimes be the soul's choice? A story told by Sarah Hinze in *The Castaways* suggests that souls on their way to birth can choose to turn back. In this case, a woman was carrying twins and enduring a difficult pregnancy. One night, while she slept, her husband had a visitation. The room became illuminated, and in the light he perceived a young man who appeared to be about twenty years old.

> The youth looked softly upon my sleeping wife. Then he spoke to me. "Dad, I have come here to tell you that my sister and I have talked together and we decided that now is not the time for both of us to come. We have decided my sister is to come first, and I will come along after a while, when the time is right."

At the next doctor visit, it was discovered that one of the twins was no longer viable. A healthy daughter was born, and a brother followed twenty-one months later. Was this a decision made by the incarnating souls, out of compassion for their mother?

Mysterious Purposes

There can sometimes be strong awareness of the soul's presence in a pregnancy that ends in miscarriage. Puzzling, perhaps—the definite connection with a child who will not be born. Perhaps something is given or exchanged that requires the physical underpinnings of pregnancy, but not the completion of birth.

African spiritual teacher Sobonfu Somé offers one possibility. She suggests that in some cases we may choose to experience miscarriage, to use the pain and surprise as a way of cracking our own psychic shell. In her view, this comes about through a cooperative agreement between the unborn soul and the mother or both parents. She says: "Sometimes there are those who want to find ways to initiate contact with, or to break through to, another dimension. It starts with the willingness of the woman or the couple, whether consciously or unconsciously, to experience something deep, profound, and life-altering. An agreement is made with beings from the other side to experience something of unknown design that will open her to the mysteries of the universe."

Or perhaps miscarriage is like an audition, trying out the fit of our energies—the prequel to a relationship that will be acted out later. In the spring of 1843, American author Nathaniel Hawthorne and his beloved wife Sophia lost their first child in miscarriage. In the journal that the couple kept together, Nathaniel wrote, "We do not feel as if our promised child were taken from us forever; but only as if his coming had been delayed for a season; and that, by-and-by, we shall welcome that very same little stranger, whom we had expected to gladden our home at an earlier period."

Miscarriage could be a time of practice at connecting soul-to-soul. Perhaps we are developing our soul sense, as we seek to navigate through threatening symptoms and save the pregnancy. We might experience an essence that we will recognize again if this soul returns:

Margaret: The complete opposite of loneliness

About five years ago, I had a dream about a friend who had died tragically. I dreamed about this friend often in the years after he died and he would tell me his experiences on the other side. In this particular dream he told me, "I met your son." He went on to describe my son, his gentle personality, dark hair and so on. At the time I was amused by the idea but was not at a place in my life where I would have considered parenthood.

Two years ago I got pregnant unexpectedly and it was the greatest joy of my life. I found out at six weeks. I enjoyed one privately blissful week where I felt the presence of my son, and then—nothing. I knew something was wrong. Rather than go to the doctor I meditated on my cervix staying closed (which it did) so that I might not lose the pregnancy.

During that blissful week, I knew I had company. The best way I can describe it is a feeling that is the complete opposite of loneliness. I wasn't lonely in my life before being pregnant. I am blessed with many loving people, but this presence elevated that blessedness infinitely. Wherever I would go and whatever I was doing, I had this encompassing sense of contentment, comfort, and peace that I had never known before or since. I felt that I belonged to the life I was carrying and the life I was carrying belonged to me. It was a truly wonderful time.

And then our connection was broken. I am not sure why this happened but I do have trust in a wisdom higher than my own and accept that the "whys" aren't mine to know right now. Once the connection was lost, I went into a complete panic and denial about the demise of the pregnancy. On some level I knew that it was not meant to be, yet I struggled to accept that reality, denying how sick I was and how much pain I was in.

As the weeks went by I got sicker and sicker and more and more desperate to hang on to something that was not meant to be. The spirit of my son was trying to leave and I just could not let him go. At night I would wake up convinced that I could hear my baby crying. Then I had a very profound dream.

I dreamed about my little boy. He was about two and a half and he was running away from me and I could not catch him; just when I would get close enough he would scoot around or under a piece of furniture. In the dream I thought, "Please, just let me see your face." When I woke up I knew this little boy was telling me to let him go, that it was not his time and my hanging on was not right.

The next day I went to the doctor and had my miscarriage diagnosed and treated with a D & C. It was the saddest period of my life and I grieved for over a year. In spite of the extreme stress, worry, and grief that I was experiencing throughout the process, I also had the experience of being accompanied by a presence that was comforting and reassuring. I have never known the depths of such sadness before, yet I always knew I was going to get through and I was going to be all right.

I am trying to conceive again and trying to be open to the signs. Last September I had another dream, where my child called me on the phone and said, "I just wanted to say hi—it is still too soon. I will see you later." Then two weeks ago I had another dream where I was out of my body watching myself about to deliver a baby. I am hoping this is an indication that the time is getting closer.

I want to share a more recent experience too. After I read the letters on your website, I was overcome by a pang of sadness for my lost son. That night before I went to bed, I asked for a visit, some contact, something to sustain me in my efforts to bring a child into this world. I found myself in a dream. I was in a department store and I was shopping for pajamas as a gift for a child that I know. Then all of a sudden I heard a little voice ask, "Will you pick me up?" and I looked down and there he was! A very beautiful and loving little boy. I finally got to see his face! I picked him up and carried him away with me. I woke up with renewed hope that I will become a mother.

A year later, Margaret reports: "We have been very busy moving over the last month. The reason for our move? The need for more bedrooms—I am eight and a half months pregnant with my little boy! And yes, he has been visiting in my dreams. He has been telling me not to worry about the birth, that he knows how to do it, that he has done it before and it will be fine." In mid-September the baby was born, "such a calm and content little boy who has a very mature spirit."

Footloose Souls?

In her book *Welcoming Spirit Home*, Sobonfu Somé describes a perspective that is quite different from our customary thinking, but nonetheless logical. She explains that in the belief of her Dagara people, a miscarriage may occur when the being who has decided to enter the womb is a "traveler," a spirit who likes to wander the galaxy rather than settling down. Such beings (*chiekuo*) are not uncommon, says Somé, adding that she herself is one of them. "Somewhere in the depths of my being," she says, "I can still remember the times my mother was pregnant with me and had to miscarry simply because I was not here to stay."

In the tradition of Somé's people, the restless soul can be persuaded to change if the community rallies around after a miscarriage and communicates with it. Each person gives a gift to the child and makes a request, such as: "On your next trip back I need you to commit to staying so we can grow together and let our spirits bloom together." Sobonfu explains that the point is to tell the soul "that miscarriage and grieving are not at all fun to be going through and you want it to stop now. You must reiterate to the spirit the significance of its being here.

When you voice your concerns it makes the spirit realize that it has to be cautious and that it can't just use the body of this woman to go back and forth between dimensions."

By acknowledging that the soul is aware and that we can effectively interact with it, the Dagara cope with loss in a pro-active manner. It is a thought-provoking contrast to the feelings of helplessness and isolation that so often accompany miscarriage. When a Dagara woman has experienced a series of miscarriages, stillbirths, or infant deaths (all escape routes for the footloose spirit), a mark may be placed on the dead child's body, in the expectation that it will show up as a birthmark when that soul returns in a new body. This might seem far-fetched, but the reincarnation research of Dr. Ian Stevenson has documented a connection between birthmarks and wounds incurred in a previous life. From her own experience, Sobonfu describes the results of her community's pragmatic approach to pregnancy loss and infant death:

> I carry a mark on my body from my former life. When I was born again, some people present at my birth had also been present at the marking of my previous body. These people performed a recognition ritual acknowledging my return. They said, "We know who you are. We see the mark we put on you the last time. This game stops now! Now that we have you in our hands, you are not going anywhere."
>
> This ritual does not guarantee that a chiekuo will not try again to slip away, but it gives the elders a chance to stay alert, keep their eyes on the baby, and work with the baby to facilitate a change in his or her pattern.
>
> I continued to try to find ways to leave this world and return to the world I knew so well, but this time each attempt resulted in doors being shut to show the determination of my people to keep me here...I was about six years old when I finally decided to put an end to the process of trying to leave. Although it was difficult for me to have to stay, my mother befriended me in a special way and made me promise to stay.

Julie, an American woman, offers a story that parallels the African concept to a remarkable degree. An added insight here is that her mother acknowledges her own participation in the series of losses, which Julie remembers instigating as a vacillating soul.

Julie K: On my way to be human

I want to talk about my decision to be born in human reality, and how as soul I and my mother vacillated back and forth, causing her to experience stillborns and early deaths.

It was very difficult for me to face, a few years ago, that I was the soul who continued to have a mind change and put the family and especially my mother through all of the yuck. However, I didn't feel the sadness and remorse until after I'd begun to grow emotionally and spiritually, and these things emerged over the years as it was time for them to come forth. At first I rejected that I was the same soul who kept halting the birth. In a very powerful dream I could no longer deny it.

When my father died at seventy-six, I took his death exceedingly hard because he was my anchor. I never doubted that my father loved me. A year after his death I felt awful. My patience and tolerance were going out the window, and as the administrator of a residential program to help alcoholics stop drinking, I needed to keep my wits about me. I finally sought help from a therapist and began to grow and grow.

I began to have spiritual awakenings and eventually they became of the metaphysical type. In therapy I learned to pay attention to my dreams. One night, thinking I was going to get up, I turned to look back and saw my body still sleeping. I felt scared, but a hand touched me and it was my mother who had herself been dead for almost two years. Then I saw my grandparents and other family and I knew that wherever I was going, I was safe. I simply relaxed and it's a good thing I did, because off and on I had more experiences like it.

I was excited, delighted, and comfortable the first time some "Beings" came in the middle of the night to get me from my bed and I followed them. For weeks before they came, my mother had popped in on me now and then only to say, "We'll be seeing you soon where we are."

It was a few days before my fortieth birthday and my fourth time with her and the others. I was told that I needed to view some of the things that happened on my way to be human. A curtain opened and I saw four of the same scene, each containing the identical woman, who was my mother in human form. She was having a baby. In the first scene I was removed as a stillborn infant. In the second, the baby lived a day or two and died. In the third scene the baby lasted a couple of weeks and died.

In the dream I felt enormous mental, emotional, and physical anguish. I wanted to run, but a loving force of light kept me in place, and I began to cry, cry and cry. I sent the thought of asking forgiveness to the soul who had been my mother. She looked very lovingly at me and sent me the thought, "I was a willing participant in the first two instances, and I understood your needs on the last time. I was glad on your fourth trip you decided to stay, for you, as soul to grow."

I shook my head accepting her forgiveness. It allowed me to forgive myself. She came over to me and we allowed our hearts to meld with each other. As a result I realized that I had as great a mother as I did a father.

The Fragrance of a Soul

Although I usually say that I had no sense of presence with my lost pregnancies, perhaps my understanding of "presence" is too narrow. At the end of my first miscarriage (devastating because I had been waiting so long for this child), I felt an unexpected peace settle over me like a gentle hand, or a refreshing rain. Two years later, just days before my daughter's birth, I was immersed in peace that lasted for hours. Looking back now over the past twenty years, I can see how unusual, for me, was my experience on those two occasions and how similar they felt. Perhaps that peace was truly a presence, the signature of my daughter's soul.

The following story goes deeper into the possibility that miscarriage leaves us with the subtle impression of a soul we shall meet again.

Lisa: An indelible imprint

When I was seventeen years old I missed my period and went to a local Planned Parenthood, scared out of my wits, to receive a pregnancy test. The test came out negative, but somehow I believed it was wrong. Despite my protests, they maintained I was not pregnant.

A month or so later I awoke with horrible pain and vaginal bleeding. I thought I was having a bad period, but the pain became so unbearable that I called my mother in tears. She intuitively knew something was wrong and rushed home to find me lying on the floor in pain. My hands and face were turning blue and the blood just kept coming. At the hospital the doctor found that I had been pregnant for fourteen weeks and was in the midst of a full-blown miscarriage.

The pregnancy and miscarriage caused severe anemia. I remember being plagued with sadness, confusion, and remorse. Thus began a haunting feeling of grief that settled over the back of my mind for many years, along with the nagging peripheral notion that I was not alone. I believe it was a boy, but does it matter?

In my experience, there is a distinct taste and smell that permeates your body when you become pregnant. Like picking up your lover's shirt and inhaling it, someone's unique chemistry has invaded your body and you can identify its distinctiveness using all of your senses. It leaves you with an indelible spiritual imprint that you carry around forever.

I am now married and thirty years old. But since that miscarriage at seventeen, I've experienced visits from this entity. Sometimes it comes to me in the form of a dream. I see the smiling face of an infant. It never says anything because the feelings speak for themselves. The face is never completely clear but the taste and smell and the feelings and lights surrounding the being have remained the same.

I'm overwhelmed with warmth during these dreams and feel the need to weep. I try and talk to it, to say how sorry I am that I couldn't keep it—I was a party teenager when I became pregnant and wasn't healthy enough to sustain a life. It just keeps smiling in a way that reassures me without the need for words.

Other times it comes to me simply as a feeling surrounding me. When I've accomplished something great and feel excitement, I feel someone "else" becoming happy and excited. I get this childish rush and literally jump for joy. When I'm sad or anxious I sense this being and it somehow encourages me to feel better. It's as if someone is holding my hand, watching over me. Someone I know and instinctively love and yearn for.

My husband and I are going to start trying for a family on my birthday in five months. We're using the time between now and then to prepare our bodies and make room in our lives for conception. And as the days draw nearer this little being seems to be coming closer and closer into the "folds" of my life. The dreams are more frequent...the radiant, smiling face surrounded by light filling me with love. The visions are becoming clearer...a tiny little firefly buzzing around above my head with anticipation. And the more excited I get at the prospect of our reunion, the more excited it becomes. It's as if it already has its suitcase packed!

Is it really possible that a soul can return to us after miscarriage and take birth in a new body? There are mothers and fathers who suspect their child is indeed the same being who was with them once before but didn't stay. Cheryl Anne Mohr has reason to believe that two of her three children are souls who made the return trip after miscarriage.

Cheryl Anne: Lost and Found

My youngest son has a very special story. You see, this beautiful little boy running around my home is the same sweet soul I lost in a miscarriage. I lost that baby at about twelve weeks, but I knew he was a boy. We chose a name for him, James Jordan; we would call him Jamey. Another thing I knew about him was that he would love to sing. I imagined him singing with the angels. My heart was broken. A few months later I found myself expecting once again, and we were blessed with our glorious firstborn son, Jon-Kyle. He was so sweet and beautiful and brought us so much joy!

When he was two years old, we conceived another child. I knew instantly that I was pregnant and that this baby would bring remarkable love and happiness to our lives. Both sonograms during the pregnancy indicated I was carrying a girl, but I knew otherwise. Thus our second son was born.

It was then that I did something very out of character. The name Jamey had been sacred to me since the loss of my first baby, yet I was compelled to call this little baby in my arms Jamey. And so we named him Jameson, and called him Jamey. I didn't really give it a lot of thought. I was so caught up with falling in love with him and enjoying motherhood!

Then one day when Jamey was two years old, he woke up from a nap in a state of total panic. "Mommy! Where is Jesus?" He was looking around the room, expecting to find Him there. He went on to tell me how much he missed God and that before he came to earth he told God how badly he wanted me to be his mommy. It was very precious, but still I hadn't put two and two together.

One day when Jamey was four, it all came together. The way he loved being a baby…he nursed for three years and savored every minute of his babyhood. I've never seen a happier baby. Every day he enjoys life more than anyone I've ever met. I liken it to a person who is on their way to the Bahamas for a vacation and the flight gets canceled. By golly, when they finally make it to the Bahamas, they're going to enjoy it all the more! Then there is the way he loves younger children. He is nurturing and protective and wants a baby brother or sister more than anything. He has the heart of a big brother. (Sadly, we lost another baby in May. Jamey told us the baby was a girl and he said her name is Rose and she'll come back. We believe him!) And then there is the way he sings!

On the day my spirit realized that this child was indeed my little Jamey, my son who had to leave, only to find his way back to me, I gave him flowers when I picked him up from preschool. It was like seeing him for the first time. I looked into his eyes and said, "I'm sorry it took me so long to realize…" He just hugged me, patted my back, and told me it was okay. I didn't have to say a word. He just knew.

Two years later, Cheryl Anne was back in touch with the moving sequel to Jamey's story:

A Winter Rose

In May of 1999 I suffered a miscarriage, which devastated my family. My two sons were so looking forward to a new baby in the family and my husband and I saw this pregnancy as a gift after working through difficulties in our marriage. Our dreams were shattered with the loss.

While I was on the examination table at my doctor's office to determine whether or not I would require a D&C, I heard a sweet, feminine voice say, "Don't be sad, when the time is right, I'll come back." I dismissed it as the voice of my own wishful thinking and sadly went on with life.

At a spiritual retreat the following autumn, I grieved in the garden of a monastery, sitting beside a single drooping pale pink rose, the last one on the bush. Then one night as I was tucking the boys in, Jamey wanted to talk about the baby. "The baby is a girl and her name is Rose," he said assuredly. "She'll come back too, just like me." While I found his sentiment to be sweet, I didn't really take his words to heart or understand how this related to the voice I heard in the doctor's office.

Several weeks later while taking a shower, the room filled with a peaceful pale pink light and I heard the voice again. "The time is right, I'm coming back." I still would not allow myself to believe such a wonderful thing and chalked it up to an overactive imagination. Soon after this, a dove began visiting my windowsill. She returned day after day. I told a friend about this and she suggested that I ask the dove what she wanted. Although I felt a bit odd doing so, I followed my friend's advice. I asked the dove why she was visiting me and laughed out loud at myself while I waited for an answer! Of course I didn't audibly hear anything, but when I got up and walked into the bathroom and caught my reflection in the mirror, I instantly knew I was pregnant. A few months later, a sonogram revealed that indeed our baby was to be a girl. We decided on the name Caroline Joy, but as my due date drew nearer I felt unsettled about the name.

During the pregnancy there seemed to be roses everywhere I turned. Complete strangers would give me roses or pictures of roses or poems about roses. One afternoon, a little girl from the neighborhood smiled and handed me a tiny rosebud. In that instant it all came together. The voice, the rose in the garden, the pale pink light, the roses, roses, roses! Jamey had been right—our Rose was coming back to us! I ran into the house to talk to my husband. I told him all the marvelous things I had been keeping to myself all those months. And then I told him we had to change the name we had chosen. We agreed her name would be Caroline Rose—our song of joy—our beautiful Rose.

Caroline Rose was born December 20, 2000.

14

Courting the Soul

○ ○

*I just completed another miscarriage—a real heart-wrencher.
The day I started bleeding, I had a visitation from a beautiful
man who sat on the edge of my bed and explained to me his
ambivalence about being a baby again and the "surrender" it
would entail.*

—*Jessica North O'Connell*

When the children we desire don't come easily, and we experience
delayed conception and pregnancy losses, many things come up for
question. We may question our worthiness to be a parent, or wonder
whether our lives and homes are enticing enough to persuade a soul to
join us. This introspective waiting time can be hard to endure, but it
can sensitize our psychic "antennae." It's a time of practice at opening
ourselves to potential children and sending out our heartfelt invitations
to them.

Teresa Robertson is a nurse-midwife who teaches people to communicate with their children-to-be, both during pregnancy and before
conception.[1] One of the aids she recommends is the baby altar. A baby
altar, Teresa explains, is a way to create within the home a "specific
energetic space" for the unborn soul. It focuses the parents' wishes, and
beams a constant welcome to the child. The baby altar has been helpful
to couples dealing with delayed conception and miscarriage. It was one

of the suggestions I offered to Janine when she wrote from South Africa, concerned about the difficulty she was experiencing in trying to have a second child.

Janine: Every day, I spent time inviting a child

I have a three-year-old toddler. Two years before he was born, I chose to abort a very ill, but alive, fetus at twelve weeks before s/he miscarried. When my son was born, I "knew" he had no connection with the other baby. However, two miscarriages later, I am wondering more and more about that first termination. Is it possible to scar a soul to the point of no longer being able to enter our world? I have enough self-insight to question the issue of guilt related to that first experience. Have I blocked his/her return? And is s/he blocking another's entrance? I cannot raise these questions with anyone in the medical fraternity; their response to our fertility issue is to advise us to be patient and consider drug therapy. But I suspect something else is going on.

I told Janine of my belief that incarnation involves a great deal of forgiveness and resilience, extending even to the circumstances of abortion. She then described how she began to work with her situation after learning about the possibility of communicating soul to soul.

In my search for inner peace, I have made progress in trying to balance "control," which has always been an issue for me. The fact that we fell pregnant so easily with our son convinced me that the same would happen again. We had the exact month planned when s/he would be born and then exactly when I could go back to studying. Ha! Have I learned a thing or two!

The first thing I have done is try to release control over another entity, but I have tried to regain control of my body, by supplementing vitamins and minerals, eating healthily, and meditating. For the moment, I have decided against medical intervention and instead have tried to relax the pressure on myself to be the perfect

woman. I have had to work on my feelings of guilt about not pro-
viding my son with a sibling, and not being able to nourish my
husband's baby.

Soon Janine had joyful news to report:

You won't believe how often I have thought of you and have
wanted to write—but kept waiting until I knew, as much as I
believed, that everything is all right. The wonderful news is that I
am expecting a baby in May. I'm now at thirty-two weeks and it
certainly is interesting how it came about.

After writing to you and reading the articles on your website, I
started doing exercises in meditation—focusing on the potential
life force that will translate into a fetus. Every day I spent time
inviting a child into my womb. Telling him/her that I had a special
place and we were ready as a family to welcome and love another
child. It was a wonderful way for me to get in touch with my
strengths as a parent and nurturer, as I was inclined always to focus
on the negatives, and to wonder whether I just wasn't good enough
to be a mother. I didn't realize these blockages existed until I
started focusing on inviting a child to become part of our unit.

Less than a month later, in September, I knew I was pregnant. I
hadn't done a test yet, but every day I would talk to my womb and
to the person I believed was growing inside me. I just knew it was a
boy and when I judged myself to be about six weeks pregnant, I
went for a scan to confirm that his heart was beating as strong as
ever.

We had decided to wait to tell my four-year-old (the fears of
miscarrying were never really absent) but one morning he walked
into our room and said he'd had a dream where a very nice old man
told him about the baby that is growing in my tummy. From then
on, he has just accepted it and sings and talks to the baby every day.
And there we were wondering how to deal with his insecurities!

The baby will probably be named Finnian, which means clear
thinking; it is a name that jumped out at us and just seemed to fit.
I have had a wonderful pregnancy, very easy, no morning sickness
at all. We seemed so ready to meet. I must say that I long to see
him and hold him, and I am starting to get a bit impatient! There

have been times when I would suddenly panic, trying to remember when last I had felt him moving, and then I would lie down on the bed and talk to him and ask him to let me know that he's okay. Within a few minutes he'd move around.

Everything went very well with the delivery and our son was born on May 15. He is truly a joy to have around and is always smiling and laughing, already wanting to talk ("googabamba"), and just wants to sit up to see everything.

A miscarriage often casts a shadow of anxiety over the next pregnancy. Jonathon and Kylie are an Australian couple who went through two losses, most traumatically a baby girl stillborn at twenty weeks. Jonathon doesn't have a strong belief in souls contacting people before birth or after death, yet it was his experience with a mysterious night-time visitor that helped Kylie confront her fear of "risking her heart" to another pregnancy. Kylie tells their story:

Jonathon and Kylie: "Mummy doesn't want me"

As you know, I lost my last baby, Kara, in August at twenty weeks. I really struggled with this—overwhelming grief and emotion. As time went on, I started to accept that I'd lost her, but it seemed almost every day I was faced with someone else's pregnancy. I have never had so many friends and acquaintances pregnant at once! I got to the point in October where I was trying to even deny the fact that pregnancy and babies existed. I was terrified that I wouldn't fall pregnant again, and my cycle was doing strange things as it settled down from losing Kara.

Jonathon and I celebrated our anniversary early in November. A couple of days later, he had a strange dream (although he's not entirely sure that it was just a dream) and he shared it with me. He thought he had heard our dogs growling and when he woke up (or kept dreaming), he saw a little girl at the end of our bed.

"I'm scared," she said. "Mummy doesn't want me." Jonathon tried to reassure her that yes, both of us want her very much, but that I was scared I might lose her again. He said she finally huffed out of the room—this would be most consistent with how I behaved as a child, I regret to say! He had the impression that she had come to be conceived.

When he shared his dream with me, it troubled me. I had to decide to have the courage to risk my heart again. I kept telling this little one how much I want her, but that I'm scared and to please be patient with me! Fortunately, both this child and I were brave and a week or two later I found out that I was pregnant.

The first few weeks after Jonathon's dream, in particular, I felt this little girl very close to me. For some reason it felt as though she was hovering just behind my head, on the right, and whispering to me. I recall a night a few days before Jonathon's dream when I was lying in bed, and saw swirling lights moving around the ceiling. It would have been about the time I conceived, I think. Around then, I also had a dream that a lady was whispering instructions to me. It seemed that I woke up and I could still hear her whispering, while at the same time she told me to go back to sleep, and that I would remember what I needed to remember when the time was right. These are all things that give me hope.

I've gone into this pregnancy with quite a different attitude to my first two. This time I keep thinking, whatever will be, will be. Maybe this baby will be born (and I dearly hope so); maybe tomorrow I'll lose this one too. Whatever happens, whether he/she lives for another day or one hundred years, I know I have nourished this baby with as much love as I can give. I keep telling the baby how much I love him/her (and for convenience I'll start calling the baby her) and want her to be part of our family.

Even after a child is born, it may be a wise practice to go on communicating with the soul, for the soul still feels the pull of its unborn freedom. We can speak our thanks and encouragement softly to the baby sleeping or drowsing at the edge of sleep. In the following story, Leigh responds to the possibility that her son may be undecided about staying:

Leigh Jarvis: A reluctant soul?

With my second child, I suffered from secondary infertility. I remember the first time I sensed Will's spirit—it was a full fifteen months before he was conceived. I was sitting in my living room watching a storm brew outside and I felt his soul ride in with the thunder. All of a sudden he was just "there."

That night I asked my husband if we could try for another baby. I could sense Will's spirit perched in a maple tree outside my bedroom window. It was as if he was watching us, trying to decide if he should come. As the months wore on and I didn't get pregnant, I became depressed because I knew he was there. He reacted by laughing at me for all my melodrama. He seemed unattached emotionally, although he obviously cared about us or he wouldn't have stuck around for fifteen months! He finally sneaked up on me in the exact month when I had decided to give up and let him go.

I had several dreams of twins and one dream of holding my baby daughter as she died, and begging people to do something for her. Late in my first month I bled heavily for a week and was told I would probably miscarry. I remained pregnant, but I wonder if someone else came with Will (moral support maybe?) but left before birth.

A psychic, with no knowledge of any of this, has since told me that Will was a reluctant soul and still at age two has not made up his mind to stay. Many people have said they were appalled that the psychic told me this. On the contrary, I am empowered by the knowledge of it. I have made my wishes known to Will and I am in awe of the sacrifice he made for me because I was in so much pain for the want of him. He is a happy though uncommunicative child; he has even been described as borderline autistic. He's not—he simply chooses not to deal with mundane, "human" nonsense. I can't blame him.

Last spring Willy pointed to that same maple tree and said, "Me, Mama…Me!" I think he remembers because he's still so young.

Kari Henley is a consultant for women on balancing work and family, sacred pregnancy and life coaching.[2] Here is Kari's story of a pregnancy that demanded commitment on more than one level. Physically precarious, the pregnancy was threatened by emotional factors as well. This is the story of how Kari and her unborn child consciously created a strong soul-bond to overcome the hazards facing them.

Kari: The Grandmother Spirit

I started this journey when I was pregnant with my son in 1994. I felt high and consumed by the experience and found it to be a time with heightened intuition and a sense of a constant dialogue and connection with my unborn. I started looking for some support, and found nothing! The only references I located were Thomas Verny's books, *The Secret Life of the Unborn Child* and *Nurturing the Unborn Child*, and *Creating a Joyful Birth Experience* by Sandra Bardsley and Lucia Capacchione. All are excellent. But frankly, I was appalled that was it!

I used to help run a training and development company and also taught and participated in women's groups around the themes of myth, ritual and various forms of feminine spirituality. I decided to combine my interests and create something for this time in my life. While it was fun and fulfilling to do, it wasn't until now in my second pregnancy that I have been captured with the subject again, and doing far more with it. Now it is feeling like my life's work for a while.

The story I am going to share about the vision of this pregnancy is all about Grandmother energy. My story is about the more mythological Native American Wise Elder Grandmothers. Living in Colorado almost all my life, I was surrounded with different types of Native influence, and became actively interested in the Lakota/Sioux. I lived at nine thousand feet in the mountains with a sweat lodge and medicine wheel at one time. I always felt drawn to and guided by this Council of ancient, wizened old women. They come to me often in visions or meditations and they are irreverent, laughing, poignant, and very real somehow.

I have gone through many personal changes this year, and the setting for this pregnancy was definitely less than planned. I separated from my husband last year and we reconciled in December.

In January I unexpectedly became pregnant. I felt conflicted and torn about my work and the time it required, and the stability of our relationship. Sure enough, at five weeks I miscarried. I felt the soul leaving and telling me it was preparing me for another.

About ten weeks later, I still hadn't started menstruating and was concerned. I had been feeling a little strange, but not what I recognized as pregnant; I assumed my hormone cycle was thrown off by the miscarriage. I went to the health food store to buy an herbal tincture to force on the period and lingered instead over the prenatal vitamins. Then I scheduled an acupuncture appointment to further bring on the cycle and something screamed inside me, "NO!" So, with a sinking feeling, I took another home pregnancy test: positive. I was incredulous. I never even menstruated after the last pregnancy and I had been using a cervical cap the whole time.

The magnitude and miracle of it all stunned me. Being someone who prides myself on my body and knowing pretty quickly when I am pregnant, this one really was an inner mystery. How could I not know I was over eleven weeks pregnant?

Next day I went to a women's gathering where they demonstrated some dancing and movement. I jumped right in and decided to dance for the baby. As I closed my eyes, put my hands on my belly and swayed to the music, I saw a group of the Grandmothers appear in my mind's eye. They were standing in a cluster and then one of them stepped forward. She looked like a Kachina dancer, all dressed up in a costume with a big headdress with dangly ribbons and her face painted white. She was a short, wizened woman as old as time. She stepped towards me and said she was volunteering to be the spirit of this child and to come in for me. To help me. To strengthen me. She also said I was going to have to invite her in if I was to keep the child.

A week later I still hadn't done the ritual I knew I was supposed to do, and felt sure my marriage wasn't going to last. I couldn't bring myself to call the child in. I was on the phone at the height of my confusion and pain in the timing of this child, and instantly I started bleeding and cramping. I had a sonogram, and they found that a three centimeter piece of the placenta had spontaneously pulled away. The viability of the pregnancy was in question and I was put on a week of bed rest.

Boy, did I feel guilty! I felt an urgency to take care of myself and really go inward about what this pregnancy meant to me. I spent a week recovering and at the end of the week it was Mother's Day. At last I felt settled and sure this was a miracle that was meant to be, and felt a deep love growing. I had the house alone and set up for my official ritual to call the spirit in.

By coincidence, a friend had just given me some Native American music, so I danced around my living room with candles lit and sage burning, focusing on myself and the baby and preparing for an inner journey together. Then I moved the candles to the end tables and lay down on the couch so I had light all around me.

I felt the group of Grandmothers come and stand all around me as if they were ancient physicians examining a patient on a table. I felt energy starting to flow in and out of my womb like a river. I had all these tumultuous thoughts and felt one Grandmother put her gnarly old hand over my eyes; and instantly I felt peace. I saw a vista before me with blue sky and beautiful mountains and started flying like a bird.

Finally near the end a song came on that is Amazing Grace translated into Cherokee. Beautiful. It was then this familiar little woman came right up to me and held my face in her hands and hugged me. Her fragility disappeared and she was as strong as the world. I sank into her and felt her sinking into me, as if our bodies were merging and melting into each other. "I am in you," she said. "I am with you. We are of one body, sharing the same blood, the same cells, the same molecules. Spinning from the same strands of DNA. I am in you."

I felt a whirling rush of energy. Microcosm to macrocosm. Felt myself spinning at the cellular level, and knew this child is a great gift and a healer for me. I felt calm, grounded and completely at peace.

Since then the pregnancy has been perfect and the doctors were amazed to discover that I never passed the piece of placenta. Instead, it simply dissolved and I have not had a single complication since. They are still talking about my case when I come in for check-ups.

My marriage is over and we are separated. Rather than being completely devastated, I do feel someone is watching over me and taking all the difficult details and handling them one by one as successive miracles. I have felt great strength in a personal way and the Sacred Pregnancy material has suddenly been received with such enthusiasm and my creative energy is at an all time high. Naturally I give a lot of credit to this amazing being.

15

Carry On

Communications from the soul during pregnancy often seem designed to calm and reassure the mother. They may even include specific suggestions for a beneficial change. In these ways, the child-to-be helps in the process of getting itself born. Sometimes a pregnant woman simply feels wrapped in a blanket of comfort and confidence. Perhaps it's a blanket woven by those calming hormones…or perhaps the child is wrapping her in its own consciousness, still lingering in the harmony of pre-existence.

Here Kari continues the story begun in the previous chapter. Throughout pregnancy she feels supported by the soul of her child, and at the time of birth the "Grandmother-spirit" makes herself known both to Kari and to her midwife friend.

Kari: Her presence was a guiding light

I consider myself a rational person. While I actively embraced the mysteries of life, and minored in Comparative Religion, I had learned that mystical experiences were things of the past and not something that fit into our modern days of cell phones, internet, and fast food. Naturally, a story of this type is not something you would tell your girlfriends over a play date! The images of this Grandmother-spirit that merged inside me were so incredible, I didn't dare speak of them aloud. Her presence served as a guiding light and a source of strength, but one I held quiet and protected.

After determining there was no peaceful outcome with my husband, I wanted to protect my baby. At six months pregnant, I moved out and we officially separated. I had been laid off from my part-time job a month before, and would go into the birth with some insurance, no paychecks, and a marriage in shambles. It was a dark time. I had my two-year-old toddler in tow as I packed all I could into my aging Volvo, and we drove off to stay with some friends and figure out what was next.

While the circumstances were devastating, I finally felt free. I knew I was carrying a girl and would not put the pregnancy in jeopardy again with undue fighting and daily tears. I was making the right choice. The Grandmother/baby inside me was giving me the strength I needed to step out, and I knew I was protecting her by getting out of a constantly stressful home life. I did not feel alone.

As I felt the steady kicking, this wise one inside of me whispered her name was Maia. A moment as clear as a bell, while my son Jeremy was outside playing. I listened. I also knew she was guiding me to meet the people I needed to help me through this transition time. As if by miracle, the marriage counselors we had been seeing knew of two other women my age who were looking for a temporary place to live. One had a little boy the exact same age as mine—and the other was a midwife.

As I approached the time of giving birth, I was growing more and more uncomfortable with the hospital where I was to stay. The caesarian section rate was high and every time I drove by the place I had a deep sense of dread. I had given birth to my son in a hospital and had a fairly normal delivery. However, I did not feel good about the birth and resented the constant rotation of nurses, the interruptions for exams, the tight fetal monitor strapped on, the drugs they talked me into taking, and the uncomfortable way they strapped my legs up and apart on the table while I tried to push Jeremy out. It did not seem right, and I did not want that again.

It seemed no coincidence I was now sharing a beautiful home with another single mom and a midwife. Marguerite was calm, clear, wise beyond her years, and loving. She had delivered babies all over the world and had just returned after a long stay in Guatemala working at a water birth center. I opened up to the intrigue and mystery of giving birth at home.

I knew I was a viable candidate. Beyond the initial scare, I was having a normal pregnancy. I was young, healthy and strong. I also realized deep inside that birth was not an emergency procedure, but the most normal and natural process in the world. What would happen if I did not have that stress of an unfamiliar and unfriendly hospital and instead could move through my contractions in my own bedroom?

I was now eight months pregnant. I knew everyone would think I had gone off the deep end: a former honors graduate, Master's degree, successful in a career, now separated, pregnant, out of a job, about to become a single mother of two, and considering a home birth...It didn't sound particularly rational. Yet, as a woman, I felt invincible. The world was not going to tell me what was right or wrong. For once, I was allowing *myself* to make all the decisions, to fully listen to the voices of instinct inside and follow them with complete trust. I knew I would not make a wrong move. Even if the path around me was littered with rubble, out of the ashes I was rebuilding my life.

After making my decision, I spoke with my obstetrician. She did not try to talk me out of it, and agreed to back me up at the hospital, should anything go wrong. I was surprised and elated. I created an elaborate birth plan and informed my family and my soon-to-be-ex-husband of my plans. Living with a midwife, I would have constant care, and a second midwife would be called in as a backup once the birth was underway. A dear friend who spent twenty years as an ER nurse planned to be there as well. If a complication came up, the hospital was only a short drive away.

I sat on the spectacular porch of my new home on a blazing afternoon of Indian summer, and looked around at all I had created, just by being willing to jump off the cliff. The house was stunning, overlooking the ocean; the boys had become friends like twins and ran around the yard. Debbie, my second roommate, had quickly become like a sister. Together the three of us had set up a loving and warm home. Three women who did not know one another a month earlier, had found each other, managed to rent one of the nicest houses on the shoreline, and blended our lives with ease. I was glowing and happy. Things were going to be all right.

It was my son who predicted my labor that night. We were horsing around with the boys until past bedtime and at long last his blond little head tumbled into bed for our customary stories and cuddling.

"Mom, Grama Lucy is going to pick me up when I wake up in the morning," he said emphatically.

"No, honey," I crooned, tucking the covers under his chin. "The baby is not coming today, but Grama will be here soon. Probably later this week."

He just smiled and settled off to sleep. He was right. By six the next morning, he would be waking up to his Grama Lucy quietly bringing him upstairs to greet his new sister.

I felt fine, with no signs of early contractions. Suddenly, at eleven, I was lying in bed and felt this huge rush washing through me. It was a feeling a second-time mother knows all too well. A big strong contraction. I was overwhelmed with the sensation and also felt my consciousness spinning inward like a vortex. Suddenly, the Grandmother's face was near to mine. I could feel her breath on my face. I had not seen her since our ceremony uniting us together six months earlier. "It is time for the One to become Two once again," she whispered to me. "And *I* will be the one pulling *you* through to the other side."

With that, another contraction came on like a thunderbolt. That seemed awfully fast.

I had a moment of reservation; should I wake up Marguerite? It would probably be hours. Boom! Deep breath, head pounding, body tightening. Okay. I would just tiptoe up and see if she was awake. A soft light under her door was suddenly as welcoming as mother's arms after skinning a knee. As soon as she saw my face, she just sighed, opened up the covers, and I crawled in like two girls at camp to talk about it. I remember laughing, "You don't get this kind of treatment at a hospital!"

I think birth is like a dance, a primal drum beat with intricate rhythms. You can either attune to the dance and it fills you with movement, or you can fight it, and it sounds like chaotic noise.

When I had contractions with the birth of my son, I remember my voice rising to this shrill kind of shriek as I fought to stay on top of the pain and bear the unbearable seconds until it was over. This time, I knew more. I was wiser. I had survived a birth and recognized the signs, I had a better idea of myself, and most of all, I was completely allowed to guide my own ship.

I relaxed and closed my eyes during the contractions. The intensity was so strong, I thought I was going to faint, yet I began to understand the sensation was actually a calling from within me. With the next contraction, I let myself completely surrender; and I began to have a vision.

I saw a scene as plain as day of my former sweat lodge up in the mountains of Colorado. It was a place of comfort and power for me, but one I had not been to in a few years. There next to the lodge, was an enormous pile of round rocks. The pile must have been eight feet high; it was formidable and imposing, yet also something I knew was for me.

And so it began. With each contraction, I would shift into a shallow breathing and fall deep into a trance. I knew each one of those stones had to be moved from the pile into a nearby fire pit. The Grandmother's voice whispered in my ear that each stone was one contraction to be moved before opening to the fire of birth.

I would then abruptly emerge out of the trance into the lull of peace between contractions. This delicate state of mind could easily have been eliminated with checking for dilation and effacement, monitoring the fetal heart rate or asking insurance questions. Luckily, I was simply given periodic massage and allowed to share my insights to a quiet, listening ear.

Now my labor had a constructive task. For almost two hours, I would slip into a contraction-trance, look at the rock pile, choose the one that was jumping out at me, and discover that each represented something. One large stone seemed to embody the power of the Eagle, as if I were given a gift of understanding that the Eagle's symbol is being able to fly to the highest reaches of the sky overhead and see the world with perspective. Another stone would whisper it was representing the qualities of Compassion; another simply held the image of someone in my family, and so on. I felt like the World itself was coming to lay gifts at my feet. The weight of the stones was so real. The cold smoothness of the rock pressed hard against my swollen belly, and cracked as it slid off my fingers into the new growing pile.

Meanwhile, Marguerite appeared to be always at my side, while she invisibly began her preparations. All I cared about was having some candles and my special music I had played when I first met the Grandmothers. I trusted her completely to do the rest.

I think if I did not have this inner dream in which to focus, I would have struggled for hours fighting my contractions. Instead, I let my body receive the maximum effect of each surge, and the labor progressed quickly. I was also experiencing the painful effects of a posterior positioning. The little one inside me preferred to lie facing up to look out at the world. This pressed our spines together, which made for many pre-term backaches and a particularly painful labor.

As if shooting out of a cannon, I emerged from my dreamy reverie of steady contractions, and into intense pain no vision could abate. I moaned for Marguerite to help me survive each one and I felt I could not do this alone. I started doubting myself to make it through. I remember Marguerite calling her backup team and telling them to hurry over now as things were moving along quicker than she expected.

Laboring on hands and knees was somehow primal and familiar, and eased the posterior pain. Meanwhile, Debbie appeared with bleary eyes and tousled blond curls to investigate the noise she heard. Her eyes flew wide at the scene and she exclaimed, "How many minutes is she?"

"Until birth?" said Marguerite. "About ten minutes, get in here!"

At that moment, I literally felt my daughter's feet pressing on the tip of my uterus and an explosion of G-force pressing down like a freight train. "I have to *push*!" I yelled in shock. Surely I was not ready for pushing! It had only been about three hours—my water hadn't even broken yet.

Debbie climbed into bed behind me and I felt another enormous push like a dolphin swimming inside of me. As Debbie watched in amazement, my entire belly contorted as the baby turned in the final moments and was now in optimal labor position. She was off my spine, and ready to emerge.

Marguerite pulled on her latex gloves to check for dilation. As she reached down to begin, my amniotic waters burst into her hands, and my daughter's head was crowning. Marguerite grabbed my hands to touch her soft hair, which soared my spirits through the stinging ring of fire as my body strained to stretch wide enough to allow her passage.

Marguerite had felt connected to my baby throughout my pregnancy and now heard Maia talking to her. She had delivered many babies before, and they did "talk to her" but not as directly as my daughter. Of Maia she has written: "She is like my daughter in some ways, and in more ways, like my Ancient One-Grandmother. She spoke to me like a person standing and leaning to my ear; I can still feel it, as if my ear were warmed by her breath, as my hands were warmed by her amniotic fluid and her slippery smooth head."

I held my baby's head while she came out, and even felt the umbilical cord. It was around her neck, yet without a thought, Marguerite gently moved it aside and with a mighty push, I felt her shoulders straining against my skin. With a final rush, she slid and poured out. A girl! She was perfect and wide-eyed and silent. She was so wise. She even looked like the old woman I had imagined her to be. Her eyes were deep black pools of primordial wisdom that acknowledged the new world around her. A moment of awe filled the room.

At last, she cried and mightily slid her way up my chest to find a nipple and latch on with instant ease. Seconds later, the room was filled in steady succession with the back-up midwife, the ER veteran nurse, my mother, and my ex-husband. I was suddenly grateful for the peace I had been given to labor without catering to other personalities, fears, concerns, and distractions. I had successfully delivered a nine pound baby in three hours flat with very little pain. My Maia had orchestrated everything perfectly. The Grandmother had arrived, and the world is blessed. Ho.

Reassurance from the Unborn Soul

The messages of encouragement that help us carry on through a stressful pregnancy can be short and to the point. In fact, it is striking how often they consist of a simple announcement such as "I'm fine" and an admonition not to worry! Hope is just one of many women who have received such a message when it was needed:

*Hope**: *"Don't cry, Mother!"*

When I was about seven months pregnant, I felt sick with some kind of infection. Even though I was keeping my weekly doctor appointments and having routine urine specimens, and even though I was in great pain, my doctor didn't detect any problems. So I was never given a prescription. I was quite worried.

One day, while crying about the problem, I saw a vision of my son (this was before sonograms so I didn't know his sex and didn't expect a boy). He looked just as he did when he became three years old—beautiful blue eyes and white-blond hair. He said, "Don't cry, Mother, everything will be okay! I'll be fine!" He was born on my birthday and although my placenta was infected, he was perfect.

Laura Shanley,[1] author of *Unassisted Childbirth*, says she definitely communicated with "something or someone" during her pregnancies. But she doesn't claim to know whether it was her unborn child, spirit guides, or her own inner wisdom that taught her how to give birth safely when an unexpected complication arose:

Laura Shanley: Instructions in a dream

When I was pregnant with my second child, Willie, I dreamed I was watching a woman giving birth. She was standing over a little plastic baby bathtub and she was catching the baby herself. I heard a voice very gently say to me, "Tell her to remember not to do too much."

"Ah ha," I remember thinking in the dream, "I don't have to do anything in this birth other than to simply let the baby come out." I knew I had inner help, as all women do, and that the birth would be easy. I decided to "deliver" the baby myself.

Several months later, I went into labor. My contractions were very mild, and what little pain I was having vanished after my water broke. Since my first baby was born right after my water broke, I took out the little bathtub and stood over it as I had seen the woman doing in the dream. A little foot appeared.

I was not expecting the baby to be breech, although a friend of mine had dreamed during my pregnancy that he saw my baby standing right-side-up inside me. As I stood there with his foot hanging out of me, I said affirmations that I was not afraid. My husband asked me if I wanted to call an ambulance but I said no. I knew in my heart that I had inner help, and if I simply followed the instructions I had been given in the dream—to give birth standing, and not do too much—my baby would be born easily.

Little by little his foot descended, and within a few minutes his other foot popped out. Suddenly something inside me said the time was right and I gave one push and guided him out by the feet. A beautiful, easy birth!

Twelve years later, I read that Michel Odent, the well-known French obstetrician, believes breech babies can be born vaginally if the woman is kept in a "standing squat" or upright position, and the attendant does nothing to interfere, if at all possible. This had been the message of the dream. Incidentally, a few days after his birth I dreamed Willie was telling me he had helped in the birth by not being afraid. All during my pregnancy I had said belief suggestions that I trusted my body and was not afraid of birth. Nor was I afraid of life. I know Willie felt my faith, and was not afraid to be born.

To be reassured by one's unborn child is a powerful gift, an affirmation that we are in this together. For Beth, the experience was transforming.

Beth: Climbing the infertility wall

I want to tell you a warm, calming, knowing story of my own. My husband and I went through three years of infertility madness. A miscarriage on Clomid, another miscarriage with Metrodin shots, a miscarriage with in vitro fertilization (we froze the remaining embryos), an ectopic pregnancy that had to be terminated with chemotherapy treatment—and finally, a successful pregnancy with Zoe.

She was conceived in June 1994 through in vitro fertilization, subsequently frozen, then thawed and implanted in February 1995, and born in October of that year. I was so afraid I would lose her too. I had spotted bleeding, had to take progesterone shots twice daily, and prayed every day.

One night, I had a dream. A child, a daughter with dark hair, called to me and said, "Mom, everything will be all right, don't worry." From that night on, I knew no matter what, everything would be all right. I ended up in the hospital a few times with problems. I developed severe gestational diabetes that required insulin injections three times a day. Zoe had to be induced two and a half weeks early because of low amniotic fluid (in essence, she was suffocating). When she was born, they whisked her away before we could hold her, and she was in the neonatal intensive care unit for three days. But she's a trouper, and she was right. Everything was okay. We went home shortly after that.

When Zoe spoke to me, she appeared as two or three years old but the size of a small baby. Her face was identical to the face we know and love today. She had dark, soft, straight hair in a page boy cut. I was slightly disappointed because I always wanted a child with curly hair, but exhilarated to know that I shouldn't worry. Well, Zoe has curly, beautiful, soft brown hair that women dream about. It's long, luxurious, and flowing—not like the dream at all. Both wishes came true. A little selfish to wish for gorgeous curly hair, but my wish came true—I truly just wanted a healthy and happy child.

I've learned to listen to my heart, intuition, and dreams because of this experience of unconditional love. I've been given a gift, my first child, Zoe (which means "life" in Greek). Six months later, we were blessed again, learning that I was pregnant with our second child, Julia. The two girls are fifteen months apart and the first year was crazy, to say the least. But I've been doubly blessed. Julia was conceived naturally with very few complications, and the girls are best friends.

I believe I went through my infertility "struggles" because I needed to appreciate life more, not take it for granted. I had always been successful prior to this in career and home life, but boy was this a great big brick wall we had to try to climb. I sabotaged my possible successes so many times because I thought I had to have it all—career and home. I was so naive. I didn't even know what "family" and "home" meant then. I was prepared to become pregnant, put my child in daycare, and return to a seventy-hour-a week full time job. Life works in mysterious ways and I believe there is a purpose for everything. We may have free choice but if we listen we won't be alone; we will always be guided for the best.

The following story is remarkable for several reasons. It suggests that a fetus as young as twenty-one weeks' gestation can act to save itself—and remember the experience years later. On the mother's part, this story illustrates that mysterious "knowing" I often hear about, whether in the form of "Everything seems normal but I just know something is wrong," or the opposite assurance that, in spite of frightening signs, everything is really all right. Perhaps this non-logical conviction is a kind of communication with the unborn soul, though it may not be recognized as such when there are no words involved.

Caitlin McKnelly: That unshakable conviction

When I was twenty weeks pregnant with my son I developed a rare condition, usually fatal for the fetus, wherein I lost all the amniotic fluid due to a tear in the membrane. About ten days after this happened, my son turned and went breech, plugging off the tear with his buttocks and permitting the fluid to re-accumulate. The position he assumed is called a single footling breech, where one leg is flexed and crossed in the usual breech position but the other one is stuck straight out.

My son is now eight years old. I have never spoken to him about the circumstances surrounding his birth, as much because I didn't think he would understand the complexities as for any other reason. However, his extended leg was contracted into that position when he was born and he could not bend his knee. This year he finally had surgery to correct this.

On a pre-surgical visit, he told the doctor an amazing tale. He said he remembered that when he was inside me, one day something happened and all of a sudden he couldn't move and he was being horribly squeezed. With a tremendous effort, he gathered all his energy and turned his body so that he could stick out his foot and push against the wall so he wouldn't be squeezed out of me, and so that he could use his body to plug off the place where the fluid was escaping. The doctor was amazed and I too was floored by this revelation from my son.

When the rupture happened, the reaction from the perinatal specialist whom my obstetrician consulted was that my only option was to abort the pregnancy. His reaction isn't as shocking as it may sound because nearly all women who have this condition miscarry anyway.

I refused to accept this verdict. I knew my baby was not only fine but that he would be born fine. I cannot tell you how I knew this, but I believed it with every ounce of my being. I had family members and friends, even my own husband, accusing me of being unrealistic and in denial. I had to find another perinatal specialist who would accept me as a patient. When I asked my obstetrician to refer me to the second doctor, he told me he felt I was being foolish but he would do what I requested.

Throughout the following weeks before my son was born I carried that unshakable conviction with me all of the time. They sonogrammed him weekly, and with every sonogram I watched him grow. He was born at thirty-six weeks, a bit premature but more than capable of a normal birth.

Looking back on the experience, the feeling I remember most is that I was not fighting *for* my baby but fighting *with* him. We were partners, and we worked hand in hand to get him into the world whole and healthy. As they were prepping me in the labor room (he was born C-section), a resident came in and told me that even if he was born alive there was still a possibility he could die from under-development of the lungs due to lack of amniotic fluid. (The fluid is essential for proper growth of a baby's lungs. It's what they use to "practice breathe" in the womb.) Rather than scaring me, it went in one ear and out the other. I still had the unshakable conviction that my son was going to be born just fine. And you know what? He was.

16

The Dialogue of Acceptance

o o o o o o o o o o o o o o o o o o o o o o o o o o o o o o o o o

It shouldn't be thought of as strange or impossible to converse with the unborn child the way we would with a mature and wise adult. Indeed, it is not the fetus we must talk to but the aware spirit.

—*Dr. Joanne Klink, Ph.D.*[1]

Stories of pre-birth communication show unborn souls taking an active role in every step of their journey to the world. There are couples who suspect their future child even had a hand in bringing them together. We've seen examples of a soul's patient courtship of its parents-to-be, and encouraging contacts both before conception and during pregnancy.

The process of working things out doesn't necessarily end when pregnancy begins. There may still be obstacles to contend with, requiring further dialogue. Even when a pregnancy is not entirely welcome, contact with the soul can help an unsure parent to embrace it.

Eidin: Not the right time to arrive

Just after I conceived my child (I knew the next day that I was pregnant because it felt like a samba band was celebrating in my body!), I had a "meeting" with the soul of my child. I was meditating and visualized walking into a room where a young man was sitting at a table. He was tall and brown-haired, and smiled slightly. I stood there and tried to explain to him that it was not the right time to arrive on the planet and that certain people would be angry and upset.

His reply was, "So?" And then I knew that we were going to be just fine. Other people's perceptions were in fact ego based, and ultimately everything was just as it was meant to be. I gave birth at home to a beautiful baby boy, knowing full well all through my pregnancy that I was to have a son. Juno is now six months old and is my joy and inspiration. Together we have already traveled thousands of miles and he is so sunny and happy that he brings delight to everyone he meets. We have been exploring the west of Ireland with him ensconced in his buggy and me with the rucksack!

I am a much better mother having known all this time that my son will one day be that confident man I met in my vision, and I will be forever grateful knowing that he chose to come through me into this world.

Claudia Griffin: "Oh, it's you!"

My story is short but even to this day, twenty-seven years later, I still feel such overwhelming joy when I remember it. I was eight months pregnant, unmarried, and living with friends far from my family. I had decided to give my baby up for adoption, and my friends and I were planning a trip to Europe after I gave birth.

It was very early in the morning when I awoke, and no one else in the house was awake yet. I lay there trying to go back to sleep, and I guess I did because I started dreaming but it didn't really feel like a dream. I "dreamed" I—my consciousness—went inside my body to where my baby was, and the instant I was there it was complete, joyous recognition!

I said, "Oh, it's you!" and that is the last coherent thought I had. I know we greeted each other lovingly and began communicating but I don't know what we said. I also had the impression that while I was giddy with excitement and in awe that this could be happening, my baby was happy but rather complacent about the whole encounter.

My son, Justin, was born a month later, and while I can't say that this event changed my decision to give him up, I am sure it had something to do with it, because as soon as I gave birth I knew I couldn't go through with the adoption.

The few people I have told this to looked at me as though they thought I was crazy, so I haven't told this story in quite a while. Thank you for allowing me to tell it again without fear of being thought "touched."

Believing that birth is "an agreement between all parties involved" (to quote the author of the next story) makes a difference in how we experience pregnancy. Like Claudia and Eidin, Cathy finds herself pregnant at what seems to be the wrong time. She responds by talking directly to the soul about her feelings.

We communicate our emotions to the unborn child whether we mean to or not. Reliving their prenatal experiences in hypnosis, people find themselves fully aware of attitudes toward them. They know not only the mother's feelings but even those of others around them. We can't hide our troubles from the child, whether they flow through hormones to the fetus or by telepathy to the soul. We can't successfully send only "positive" messages. The practical approach, then, is to lay our emotional cards on the table and communicate as equals with the soul.

In an unusual book titled *Lovestart: Pre-Birth Bonding*, Eve Marnie proposes that an expectant parent can share her whole life with the unborn child. She deals realistically with the stress and ambivalent feelings that are normal in pregnancy. "When you are feeling stressed," she says, "keep talking to your baby and keep sharing your life." This approach seems wiser than trying to communicate only sweetness and light—an ideal that might cause you to withdraw from the conversation when sweetness and light are out of reach. Marnie explains: "It is the spirit, the divine intelligence…with whom you are making contact. What else could it be when we speak of a being six weeks after conception?…Be honest with your baby. You cannot fool your own mind and you cannot fool another part of the universal one-mind."[2]

Cathy's story puts pre-birth communication into the longer time frame of several pregnancies and births. Along the way, it introduces a mystery that we'll explore in later chapters: the confusing experience of having expectations that don't come true.

Cathy: Living with Soul Communication

I have a son and a daughter from my previous marriage. I knew a couple of months before I became pregnant with my son that it was time for both children to be born. I didn't have a dream or a vision or anything like that; it was just that I felt these two beings around me all the time. They "told" me (not in words, but in a certain knowingness) that it was time for them to be born. I knew what they would look like, their personalities and differences. Today, their looks and personalities are exactly as was made known to me.

In *Soul Trek*, one mother described having a presence hovering about her and she mentioned that it always seemed to be up and to the right. When I read that, I felt a chill run through my body—I remember that feeling exactly from the pre-birth contact with my children! It was as though you were always looking up and slightly to the right, trying to catch a glimpse of whoever was there.

Now I am re-married to the man of my dreams and we are expecting our first child in April. When I was in my teens, I had another "being" who came and stayed around me for a while and I knew he was to be my son someday. I knew he had dark hair and dark eyes (which much resembles my husband now) and for some reason, he needed me to be his mother. Strangely enough, when my first son was born, although I loved him enormously, I knew he was not that being.

During this pregnancy, I have had very little contact with the soul of this new baby. It feels as if he has been away finishing things up or preparing things. However, in the first trimester our family was going through a lot of tribulations and nothing seemed to be going right. My husband and I weren't even sure whether having another child was the right thing to do at the time. One day I was very depressed and upset with our situation and I mentally told the baby, "It's okay if you want out of this. It's still early in the pregnancy and you can leave if you want to."

The next morning I woke up to some spotting! I was convinced I was going to miscarry and was devastated and felt guilty and grief-stricken. It made me realize how very much I did want this baby. At the same time, I felt as though the soul of this child knew that being born was an agreement between the two of us, and I think he respected my feelings enough to leave if it wasn't right.

I went straight to bed to rest and tried telling this baby how much I did want him to stay and how much I loved him already. The spotting went away and the pregnancy has been perfectly normal. I am anxiously awaiting the birth of this baby to see if this is the same soul I met so many years ago.

About a week before my due date, my husband and I were sitting in our office talking about our future and the baby and how frustrated we were with our lives—we were just ready to give up—when we both smelled the sweet fragrance of flowers. I have always believed this signaled that angels were near, and we took it as a sign of hope.

That night as we lay in bed, I felt the soul of this baby enter my body. Up until this time, I had never really felt any communication with this soul. It just seemed to be near sometimes but most often away. The feeling was that of a bright presence that slowly approached from the left and settled into my body. When I told my husband the next morning, he said he had been dreaming about our baby. He was sitting on the couch with a little boy of about five years old and they were looking through photo albums and he was telling this little boy all about other members of the family.

We planned a water birth at home with our midwife and her apprentices in attendance, which was an incredibly empowering experience in itself. When I finally pushed the baby out into the warm water of the birthing pool and my husband lifted that warm, wet body onto my abdomen, the midwife asked my husband what we had. You can imagine my amazement when he announced, "It's a girl!" All this time I was so absolutely certain this baby would be a boy! Of course we fell in love with her immediately. But at the same time, I felt there was a baby missing and a deep sadness, as though a baby had died.

As the days went past, my husband and I both came to the conclusion that we were grieving for a child who had never been born. It took us a while to get through that emotion, and of course our little Kelley Lynne was more than we had ever dreamed of. We love her so much!

There are a few interesting factors. The placenta was very large, and the midwife made a comment about "a double walled membrane," which makes me wonder if there were supposed to be two babies. I had some spotting early in my pregnancy. I wonder if perhaps one of the babies chose to leave at that time. Also, my husband and I are both in the later years of our baby-making days and I know if this baby had been a boy, we would have stopped completely. Maybe this little girl wanted to make sure she was born, too! Now we talk about maybe having one more. Who knows?

July 2000...We have had another baby, an unexpected pregnancy when Kelley was nine months old. When I found out I was pregnant the second time, it was again a very stressful period in our lives. My husband and I were going through some difficulties in resolving our "spiritual" differences (he is Christian; my beliefs are a little more expansive) and even though I really wanted to have another child some day, I had decided I didn't want to bring another child into such a relationship.

I was absolutely devastated by the news that I was pregnant. All our disharmony, coupled with the fact that Kelley was still such a baby, had me feeling out of control. After a good long cry, I sat down and firmly told this baby it was not wanted at this time, thank you, and I was ready for it to leave. I felt as though this child was not taking my feelings into consideration, and because I believe birth is an agreement between all parties involved, I was really angry. I even took extra vitamin C and ginger tea to encourage the baby to leave.

But for some reason, I felt this baby had things under control and figured out. I got a very distinct "It's okay—everything will be all right" message, almost as if the baby were trying to reassure me. And it was not budging or going anywhere!

Not long after, my husband and I both received guidance not to worry about each other's spiritual side and were able to let go of all our perceived differences. We are lucky to be one of the few couples we know who truly love each other! And I was able to accept the fact that we were having another baby.

Since I had always felt that the little soul who communicated with me when I was a teenager would someday be my son, you would assume that I thought this baby would be the one. But I didn't. This was someone new. My husband and I never picked out names for her until she was born. We both knew she would name herself, and although we would have liked to have a boy, I think we both just knew it would be another girl. When I was pregnant with Kelley I felt that she wasn't around very often, but would check in with me and her developing physical form. This baby was present from the beginning. I never felt the presence leave.

Corinne Victoria was a true post-date baby. She and I worked together during labor and communicated continuously. At a certain point, I felt she needed to be born as quickly as possible. My water broke and we discovered it was meconium stained (a sign of fetal distress). All of a sudden, it was as if my body and the baby went into high gear and she arrived after the next two "expansions."

Of course, we all fell in love with her immediately. I felt very comfortable with her, as if she had been an old friend, and it didn't take me a few days to discover who she was, as it did with Kelley. I can't imagine what life would have been like if she hadn't decided to stay.

I have come to realize that I did invite her to live with us, unconscious as it might have been. I am discovering that what we think is what manifests in our lives, particularly in very energetic situations! And I have to watch my thoughts when my husband and I are being intimate; I can actually feel another soul just waiting in the wings, waiting for me to give intent to our purpose and open the doors for another baby. It's almost an unsettling feeling at times.

Sometimes I feel an overwhelming sadness when I realize that I will never be the mother of the soul who visited me when I was young. At these times, a chill envelops my body, and I can feel the presence of this entity. Things just did not work out for us in this lifetime and I have encouraged this soul to find someone else who can allow him the opportunity to be in this plane.

17

Soul and Body

The fascinating thing about babies is that they seem quite able to think and know things long before they can demonstrate this in conventional language. This makes the new findings on direct communication with babies—telepathy, really—such a significant breakthrough in understanding the infant mind.

—David Chamberlain, Ph.D., *personal communication*

Jenny Wade, Ph.D., is a professor at the Institute of Transpersonal Psychology and author (among other works) of an article whose title tells the whole story of this chapter. In "Two Voices From the Womb: Evidence for a Physically Transcendent and a Cellular Source of Fetal Consciousness," Dr Wade writes:

> The data strongly suggest that two sources of consciousness exist: One state of consciousness that is tied to the physiological development of the fetal body, especially the central nervous system; and another that appears to function relatively independent of the body…When it can be separated from its sensations of the body, the transcendent source appears to be fully mature and insightful…It is characterized by a sense of self but relatively little ego, and it seems to understand the reactions of others with compassion rather than through the lens of ego defense structures.

Two sources of consciousness: here is an idea that supports the logic of pre-birth communication, for it seems reasonable that the source "relatively independent of the body" can interact with other souls. Dual consciousness explains why communication often decreases after conception, or fades in the later months of pregnancy as birth approaches. It is as though the transcendent source gradually steps back while the fetal awareness grows. Such was June's* experience during her pregnancy:

> This child communicated many things to me about herself and gave me advice as to the best food to eat for the baby, what vitamins to take and so on. I had been a vegetarian for about a year, but she told me I needed to eat red meat. As it turned out, I had become underweight and very weak on the vegetarian diet. She guided me through my pregnancy as to what to do and not do for the best interests of us both. I was in such an expanded state of awareness.
>
> Close to the eighth month, there was a shift. I started feeling disconnected and very sad and alone as if someone dear to me had left me. I panicked! I started desperately asking what was wrong. Unfortunately, as I learned, when you get emotional and ungrounded you can't communicate properly. She finally got through to me that she was not going to be with me in the same way any more; she was going to join her body. This was all very new and strange for me. She had to stay in her body from now on and couldn't be out and about as before. She had to prepare for birth.

What Dr Wade terms a transcendent source of consciousness is what I call the soul. She proposes that the soul consciousness is present and active as early as conception, throughout pregnancy, and for a few days postpartum. After that, it becomes more or less eclipsed by the "brain-based sources of awareness," but young children can still access soul consciousness fairly easily up to about age five. (In later chapters, we'll see many examples of this wondrous ability.)

Nowadays, expectant parents are encouraged to communicate with their unborn child, but the focus is often all on the fetus, on stimulating the senses and giving the brain a head start. I am concerned that some plans to "begin educating your baby in the womb" carry a subtle message of parental anxiety and pressure to perform, to be a "gifted" child. Prenatal stimulation needs to be offered gently, with respect for the mystery of unborn consciousness and its rhythms of sleeping, dreaming, and remembering.

But our approach is different when we are speaking to the soul. We can take a hint from a book that is not as well known as it deserves to be, *Diary of an Unborn Child*. Mirabelle Coudris, a young Austrian woman, felt "a strong urge to listen in to the baby" during her fifth month of pregnancy. Over the following weeks she transcribed a series of messages, ranging from details of life in the womb to observations of the outer world. If these are truly communications from the soul, they are illuminating. The unborn child seems to perceive the outside world both directly and telepathically through the mother's mind, and his comments about it are a blend of innocence and wisdom. He says that he often sees images of his mother's thoughts, "but I do not always know what this picture is or means, unless you explain it to me." Mirabelle hears her child say:

> There are several ways for us little ones to make contact. One is through the embryo. Everything which goes on in this tiny little body is experienced. But don't think that that is all!…What you perhaps do not know is that what this body is helping to produce, namely the being of the human-to-come, was always there and always will be! Only, its experience alters its personality—as when after a profound experience you are no longer the same. A similar thing happens to an embryo as happens to you in sleep. It lives without a body, set free, living in the spirit.[1]

The Wide-Open Awareness of the Newborn

If the transcendent source is still very present at birth and for a while afterwards, do we see evidence of it in new babies? Surely, many people have felt that a wise, ancient being gazes out at them from newborn eyes. Observations from a variety of sources testify to the unusual awareness that infants display:

A mother:

When Daniel popped out and they handed him to me I had the overwhelming impression that he knew just where he was. When we went to the recovery room and Sam, who was then almost seven years old, joined us, I got a second strong impression that he and Daniel were already acquainted. It sounds very simple but really I would say it has changed my life.

A Dutch maternity nurse:

I come into contact with many newborn babies. It is perfectly true that when they cry and I tell them they can do it, and it is not so bad here, they look at me then with big round eyes, quiet down and "talk" to me in eye-language.[2]

Rhodora, a pediatrician:

I usually talk to my newborn patients in the nursery, and I find that when I tell them to put their tongues out or blink or raise their hands or even wave "bye," they do it most times. What shocks me is when I haven't yet said it, and they start to put their tongue out, or show their dimples, or even smile. Sometimes I make a funny remark, and they start to laugh! I try not to show any expression when asking them to smile or blink their eyes or put out their tongues. I do know that newborn babies imitate facial expressions, so I just talk to them. They seem to understand anyway.

A psychoanalyst:

Dr. Myriam Szejer is a classically-trained Freudian analyst who "talks to babies." She believes the unconscious is totally open in the first few days after birth, as well as during gestation. For ten years Dr. Szejer has been working with obstetric and pediatric staff at a large Parisian hospital, using her "psychoanalytic cure with babies." She is called in to see infants exhibiting all sorts of symptoms that can be translated as suffering. After gathering available information about the baby's gestation and birth, she lovingly tells the baby his/her story. After one or two sessions, the stressful symptoms disappear. Dr. Szejer says, "For an analyst to work during these days, it is much more valuable than ten years of analysis on the couch."

David Chamberlain, Ph.D.:

The view of life presented by babies at birth is an intriguing and mystical one of complete persons in little bodies knowing many things: they are frustrated that they cannot yet make their bodies work the way they'd like; they know what they need and whom they can trust; they evaluate the motivations of doctors; they perceive the psychological flaws in standard medical births; they point out virtues or weaknesses of parents; and they recognize the special needs of their siblings.

Hypnotherapist Helen Wambach, describing the experiences of people regressed to their birth:

Many subjects reported that the onrush of physical sensations on emerging from the birth canal was disturbing and very unpleasant. Apparently the soul exists in a quite different environment in the between-life state. The physical senses bring so much vivid input that the soul feels almost "drowned" in light, cold air, sounds. Surprising to me was the frequent report that the newborn infant feels cut off, diminished, alone compared to the between-life state. To be alive in a body is to be alone and unconnected. Perhaps we are alive to learn to break through the screen of the senses, to experience while in a body the transcendent self we truly are.

The Mystery of Individuality

To explore a little further, we may ask—how transcendent is the soul? It goes beyond the boundaries of the body; does it also transcend the boundaries of separate selfhood? Is soul an individual being or a shared field of consciousness?

The mystery of selfhood deepens when we discover that we can experience memories belonging to other people whom we could not "logically" have been, such as our own parents. This brings us to ask whether memories can even be said to belong to individual persons!

Now and then we come across a story so startling that our whole idea of reality has to shift to accommodate it. The writings of Stanislav Grof provide an abundance of such mind-expanding moments. This bold researcher of altered states relates the experience of Nadja, a fifty-year-old psychologist who (while on LSD) relived an episode of her own mother's early childhood.[3]

"Suddenly she was her mother at the age of three or four. The year was 1902 and she was dressed in a starched, fussy dress...hiding under a staircase. She felt frightened and lonely, painfully aware that something terrible had just happened. She realized that only moments before she had said something very bad, had been reprimanded, and someone had roughly put a hand over her mouth." From her hiding place, Nadja could see her aunts, uncles, and cousins sitting on the porch, unaware of her misery. She felt deeply ashamed, overwhelmed by her failure to please the adults with their incomprehensible demands.

Nadja was able to check this scene with her mother, relating it as a dream because she knew her mother would not approve of LSD. Quickly, her mother took up the story and confirmed the details exactly as Nadja had experienced them.

Where does one person end and another begin? If we can remember each other's memories in this way, the borders are fuzzy indeed. An experience like Nadja's implies that we are connected—more than connected—and yet we also seem to be individuals. It reminds me of a powerful description of pre-existence, from a soul memory yet to come in a later chapter: "I was a part of everything and everything was a part of me. I was aware of the connection that flowed through me to all life and all forms of life. Although I was a part of the 'all,' I was still uniquely 'me.'"

Perhaps that paradoxical unborn reality still prevails in this world, revealing itself from time to time in boundary-breaking experiences and moments of soul communion.

18

Abortion

If life is an adventure of immortal souls that exist before and after the term of their physical bodies, how does abortion fit into the picture? From this perspective, relations between souls take on new and enduring importance. I've found that the soul perspective can be used to argue either side of the abortion issue, but it can also point the way to a possible alternative, a gentler way of disengaging when circumstances require it.

Without a Name

Sweet black-haired child
you did not slip away
but were wrenched
as your mother
resisted resisting
breathing
pretending there was nothing
to do in life
but to look at the blueandgreen
plastic mobile,
pictures of human reproductive systems
muscles and tubes.

Sucked away
Unseen

chips of blue and green
swirling overhead.

Left alone
the knees tremble
the tears trickle into the ears

Will you come again,
little spirit?
Is there such generosity
in the universe?

Are you wondering
why this body embraced you?
Why it drank you up
with such a thirst for child...

...or was it you?
wandering around the stratosphere
in search of a warm nest?
Did you fly by our house
one afternoon
of custom-made lovemaking
when all of our windows
were open to new life.

To say that it was not the right time
is scarcely blanket enough
to warm the cold
that dangles between us.

—Anita

"Is there such generosity in the universe?" The answer seems to be Yes; such generosity exists and the spirit can return even after abortion. There are stories that speak of the soul's resilience and its ability to choose a new entryway when one option is denied. But some experiences reveal that abortion, or even the threat of abortion, can leave lasting traumatic memories.

Marilyn: Remembering the threat

Throughout my youth I had a terror of being rejected. I became a Christian, and this phobia was one of the first things I began to deal with. During my dealings with it according to the scriptures, I had a flashback to the moment of its origin. I saw dim shadows and heard my parents arguing. I heard my father's voice tell my mother, "Then, you'll have to get rid of it!" At that moment, I felt (re-felt) a zinging sensation, like an electrical impulse, enter me and a feeling like terror react in me.

I immediately went to my mother and asked if there had been a time when she was pregnant with me that she had discussed aborting me with my father. She looked astounded and told me there had been such a time, when the doctor told her she might not live if she continued the pregnancy due to her Rh factor complication. She asked me how I had known, and I told her I had suddenly remembered it.

A Canadian therapist describes the experience of one of her clients:

At the age of seventeen, Sue* had an abortion without consulting her parents. Afterwards she felt very remorseful and came in for therapy in which we worked on the grief for what she had done. A year later when finding herself pregnant again, she came in to see me and I took her into hypnosis where she could talk to her baby. She saw a pink bundle and held the baby and talked to her. The baby said she wanted to be born, and Sue felt a strong soul connection with her this time. She went on to have the baby girl and kept her with the help of her parents.

When the little girl was about three, Sue had to go into the hospital with an allergic reaction to something she had ingested. The grandmother took the child in to visit her, but when the little girl saw her mother in the hospital bed, she started screaming and had to be taken out of the building. When asked why she was so upset, the child replied, "I drowned in that hospital."

Carol Bowman is a pioneering researcher whose work focuses on children's memories of past lives. She too has encountered cases of a soul apparently returning to the same mother after miscarriage, still-birth, or abortion. Says Carol, "It's never too late for a mother to apologize to a soul and explain what happened—even if the dialogue is with a soul who has returned to her as another child." In her book *Return From Heaven* she tells the story of a Texas mother whose three-year-old son Joel gave her a remarkable gift.[1] As they drove home from preschool one day, Joel was quietly coloring while the radio broadcast an abortion debate. Suddenly Joel piped up, "Abortion is wrong." His mother, startled by his apparent understanding and not wanting him to learn to judge so quickly, explained: "Joel, abortion is a woman's choice. When I was sixteen I made a mistake and had to have an abortion. I always felt sad about that, but I did what I felt I had to do at the time."

She wasn't sure whether Joel really understood what she said, but then in a matter-of-fact way, without even lifting his head from his coloring book, the little boy remarked, "Don't worry, Mommy. That was me. I just went back to heaven and waited for you." His calm assurance gave his mother a sense of peace that had been missing in her life since her teenage years.

The Paradox of Levels

It is puzzling that some children talk serenely about abortion memories, while others express fear lasting across death and rebirth. The difference might lie in the level of communication before abortion, the method employed, or the soul's degree of identification with the fetal body at that point. But this puzzle suggests to me that a simple duality of soul and body cannot explain the whole spectrum of awareness.

There are complexities of experience that make sense only if we think of consciousness as many-layered, or like a lens that can focus at any depth of an infinite field. Some of the visitations from future children are so filled with what I can only call spiritual presence and wisdom, that we have to suppose we exist on more than one level of knowing. Perhaps at one level we are aware of the "big picture" and are able to foresee the probability of events such as abortion or abandonment, while on another level we have to live the experiences, down and dirty, with no understanding at all.

The paradox reminds me of the puzzle of "death trauma." When people are regressed to past life memories and recall their death, they find that death itself is blissful and perfectly safe. Yet according to reincarnation research, many of us are born with aversion and phobias around the circumstances that led up to a death. Knowing, deep within ourselves, that death was all right somehow does not erase the fear associated with it. Fear seems to be held in an emotional template and carried from body to body.

But strangely enough, consciously recalling a former death *can* relieve fear in our present life. David Chamberlain describes the case of a woman who suffered lifelong panic attacks and insomnia.[2] Through hypnotherapy, she discovered that she had endured an abortion attempt in the womb, which her twin sister had not survived. The attack upon herself, then witnessing the death and disintegration of her sister's body, left her "swimming in anxiety" as Chamberlain aptly puts it. Her fears dissolved after returning in hypnosis to a past death experience of her own, where she discovered "a luminous realm of safety and love where all knowledge was immediately available to her." As Dr. Chamberlain remarks, "This was an astonishing new idea of death." Of course, it is a familiar scene from soul memories of pre-existence.

Talking It Over

If abortion is the choice, can we soften the trauma by communicating with the soul and explaining the circumstances that led to the decision? In the following story, a mother finds that a telepathic connection seems to change the experience for both herself and the unborn soul.

In December of 1997, my husband of four months and I decided we would wait a while longer before trying to have children. We had compelling reasons for needing at least another six months before we would be ready to have a child. Unfortunately, having made that decision, I became pregnant the following month.

My husband and I wanted very much to have children. In fact, we are both only children and we wanted to have more than one child. It was extraordinarily difficult for us to decide what was the right thing to do. We knew it would be very hard for us to have a baby at that time but we wanted this child so much.

While we were considering the options, we went to church one Sunday morning. The minister led the congregation through a guided meditation. During that meditation, with no conscious intention to do so, I found myself visiting my womb and talking to that tiny, beautiful baby. There would have been no way to tell at that early stage of pregnancy, but I was certain it was a girl. I told her of our situation, why the timing was so difficult, how very much we loved her and wanted her and how painful it was to consider asking her to go and come back another time.

Though there were no "words" from her, I felt from her a tremendous sense of peace and understanding. She nodded slowly and deliberately and closed her eyes. At that moment, I rejoined the outside world with a profound sense of relief to go along with my sadness: she understood and would not feel unloved or unwanted. I did my grieving during the time between that morning and the appointment to terminate the pregnancy. Though I was sad after the procedure, I believe her soul had left already.

In August, we were ready to try to get pregnant. We conceived on the first try and I was absolutely certain this child was the same soul. My husband was certain it was a boy, and a different soul. Well, at ten weeks we had a sonogram and discovered there were two babies! In December, we learned we were having a girl *and* a boy so we were both right. My babies were born in April and they are the greatest gift I could ever imagine receiving.

Sometimes it is the unborn soul who reaches back with compassion to comfort the mother. The bond between them may still come to be realized in another way, as Natalie's story reveals:

Natalie: Reassurance from the soul

In the mid-seventies, I became pregnant for the ninth time. I had seven children and had miscarried once. I was in complete unity with myself that I could not bear another child. Everything in me said, No! I arranged for an abortion and a tubal ligation.

After the surgery, which required a hospital stay of three days, I began to recover nicely. On the final night of my hospitalization, I had a short, vivid dream in which a child's voice said, "For you, this is a big deal, but for me, it's nothing at all! I'll be born somewhere else." Gleeful laughter followed, the laughter of a child. I woke feeling healed in a profound sense. I have never forgotten the dream nor the sound of the laughter.

Nineteen years later, as I sat in my living room reading, I heard the voices of my daughter and Nils*, our Danish foreign exchange student, talking upstairs. Suddenly, Nils laughed and the hair on the back of my neck stood up. It was the laughter I had dreamed so many years ago!

Nils had come to our house by a fluke, chosen by us only because he played the organ and we had an unused one. He had originally been placed with another family, but something prevented them from taking him and our application had been misplaced by the agency and gone unfilled. When we met his plane from Denmark, I had no sense of meeting a stranger and felt I had always known him. During his year with us, we had a connection which seems to us absolute, like mother/child. His birthday pretty well coincides with when my baby would have been born.

Nils has visited us several times since he lived with us. He spent last Christmas here and is accepted by my children and grandchildren as another "brother" or "uncle." As for me, I'm profoundly thankful for the experience. The truth I know in my heart is that Nils is the incarnate soul of the baby I didn't have. My dream was one of grace, and his appearance in my life has deepened my understanding of the interconnectedness of all life.

Soul Communication: An Alternative?

Jane English is a writer, publisher, and photographer, with a Ph.D. in physics. She maintains the website Cesarean Voices "by, for, and about cesarean born people." In her book *Fingers Pointing to the Moon*, Jane English offers an approach to abortion that goes beyond the either-or standoff of the abortion debate:

> The transcendence perspective on abortion came to me when two women friends of mine happened to be visiting me in my apartment in Mendocino at the same time. As I sat there listening they discovered that each of them had had an unwanted pregnancy, and both had come, in deep meditation and with a small supportive circles of friends, to what they felt was true communication with their unborn child. The women had communicated both their love for the child and the fact of not being able to give the child a good home, physically and emotionally, at that particular time. Each said they had felt their child understood and agreed to leave. Both women had had spontaneous miscarriages the following day.
>
> By transcending conventional assumptions about the nature of human identity, especially that of unborn children, these women had simultaneously been truly pro-choice, respecting their own needs, and truly pro-life, respecting the unborn child as a sentient being. It is important to note that both of these women were psychologists who also had years of experience with meditation. We should not expect that a young teenager who is pregnant would, in a culture that sorely neglects training in inner practices, be able to communicate so well with the child. Though some might be able to do it with only the support of knowing such communication is possible.
>
> What these two women accomplished can, however, serve to broaden our perspective on abortion. It can be a goal towards which we as a culture can work. With this path as an additional possibility the intensity of the abortion conflict can be greatly lessened.

Dr. Gladys Taylor McGarey, M.D., physician and author, acknowledges that the unborn soul participates in all the phases of birth. She looks at abortion from the viewpoint of the child soul, which she maintains is aware and telepathic and has some power of choice. "In all the struggles between the pro-choice and pro-life factions," she says, "no one seemed interested in what the child thought." Based on her medical experience as well as her philosophy, Dr. McGarey agrees with Jane English that in some cases communication offers an alternative to abortion.

In one instance, a young woman was facing an untimely pregnancy but did not wish to have a medical abortion. She made a practice of talking to the child soul, suggesting it would be better for him to move on, yet leaving the choice to him. One night, she was able to move her consciousness down to her uterus. She recalls, "It felt like a cavernous, secure shelter. In a rather suspended yet elevated space, this soul and I had some serious communication. It felt completely natural. I explained that it wasn't the right time for me to become a mother. With love I let him know that it had nothing to do with him. I urged him to find another mother." The following day, she spontaneously miscarried.[3]

Ultimate Generosity: Soul Returning

Theresa Danna, M.P.W., pioneer researcher of pre-birth communication, has allowed me to share a story given to her by a California mother:

> In 1979 I was single, pregnant, and opted for an abortion. Within forty-eight hours I became seriously ill and was hospitalized for two weeks with a massive uterine infection. My physician told me it would be highly unlikely that I could ever again conceive a child. Of course I was devastated and consumed with guilt and self-loathing.
>
> In 1980 I met and married a wonderful man. I was taking birth control pills at that time, not for their intended purpose, but

because the infection had messed up my cycles so severely that they needed to be artificially induced. In June of that year I had a strange dream. My husband and I had just made love and I was drifting off into a sleep that was very vivid in its imagery. It was like I was still awake and aware that I was in my bed, yet I was an active participant in my subconscious "movie."

In the dream movie, my husband and I had just made love outdoors on the beautiful green, grassy, rolling hillside. He lay beside me dozing, and I was on my back looking into a beautiful crystal blue sky, feeling the warm sun, smelling summer on the breeze, listening to the birds and bugs. Suddenly, a small, blond child leaned over from behind me and kissed me on the forehead. It was so startling and the physical sensation so intense that I jerked wide awake instantly.

A few days later I was similarly jerked from a deep and seemingly dreamless sleep, by an external voice that was quite loud. It said, "This time you won't get rid of me." I did not take my pill that morning, and went to the doctor that afternoon. The following March, my beautiful blond daughter was born. Seven years later we were blessed with another miracle...our son.

19

Jilly's Story

Jilly is in her mid-thirties and has three children. Due to some complicated life circumstances, she has also had several abortions. Her experiences during and after her last abortion led her to create a website to provide support and comfort to all women after an abortion,[1] and opened her eyes to the reality of soul survival.

Jilly's story illuminates many ideas: children's awareness of their siblings whether born or unborn; connections to grandparents, even the ones we didn't specially bond with during their lives; and the acceptance and flexibility that grace our relationships.

> She told me her name was Lily when I was about two weeks pregnant. I heard her say to me, in my head, "I'm Lily." I remember being kind of stunned, and thought I was hearing things. I had been on two forms of birth control, and was carefully trying to avoid pregnancy. But my birth control failed, and I found myself pregnant.
>
> Lily was not born, because I had serious health problems along with some other complicated situations in my life, and I chose to have an abortion at eight weeks into the pregnancy. Even though I had made the right choice for my life and for my three children who were already here, I was devastated, depressed, and grief-stricken afterwards. I had serious trouble coping, and the first healing help was when I felt a connection with Lily and when I saw her in a dream, the night I was trying once again to kill myself.
>
> It was the first week of June; the abortion had been on May 24th. I dragged myself to the bathroom, took out all the pills I had,

lined them up on the sink and pondered them, wondering if they would be enough. I was dully afraid of winding up in the hospital with some kind of half done job—afraid of not being able to do it right—afraid of being a half-aware vegetable or something. And I heard a voice just float through the air, like some kind of psychic echo, that said, "Not yet…" I didn't even really think much about it, but just sighed and put the pills back in the medicine cabinet, and slumped back downstairs to bed. Then I fell asleep and had "the dream."

In my dream I was swimming in the water by a pier, crying. There was fog all around the surface of the water and fog on the pier. Something made me look up onto the pier, and I saw the fog at the far end lift a bit, and two shadowy figures emerged—a tall one and a short one. I stopped crying as I watched them. The figures had a halo of glowing light around them, a kind of shimmering aura. I saw the tall one hang back and noticed it was an older woman, and the short one came forward.

As she came closer, I could see it was a young girl of about six, with long brown hair parted on the side and big brown eyes. She said to me, "I'm Lily," and instantly I burst into tears. And she said, "It's okay."

"Okay? How can it be okay?" I exclaimed. "Look what I did to you! I didn't even give you a chance at life!" She was about three or four feet from me, and looked very real, even with that shimmery effect of light around her, but I could not reach up out of the water to her, and I knew somehow that I could not get on the pier. So I cried, and looked up at her.

She had such a look of compassion on her face, but then she shook her head at me and said, "It's wrong to try and cross over before your time." I put my head down and said, "I don't deserve to live, after what I did to you." Then she replied, "I knew what was going to happen even before we started down this path. I was not attached to the physical manifestation yet, and could move in and out at will. And I knew it would happen, it was meant to be, and holds a purpose for your life."

I looked at her in confusion and asked, "A purpose?" And then I abruptly switched subjects and asked her, "Why are you six? You shouldn't be six yet." She replied, "We are all ageless, and I appear as six because this is a comfortable age for you to see me as." I floated there in the water, trying to digest this, and cried a few more short sobs. She looked at me again, then held out her arms and said, "I don't need to forgive you, there is nothing to forgive. I love you with all my soul, and will see you and talk to you again."

During this dream, all the talking was done telepathically—her mouth never opened, and the words were never spoken through her mouth, yet I could hear them as clear as a bell. My talking also was telepathic, I did not physically speak either. I remember thinking how strange this was at the time, yet also so completely natural and normal that we were communicating this way.

Suddenly I noticed that the older woman had moved up beside her on the pier. I could tell then that the woman was my maternal grandmother, who had died six years ago. I remember being surprised in my dream, because I was not especially close with this grandmother, and if I were going to subconsciously choose a person to be taking care of my child in Heaven, it would not have been she; instead it would have been a very close friend who had passed on.

My grandmother did not speak, but acknowledged my presence with a short nod, then reached out and took Lily's hand, and turned to walk her back to the light at the end of the pier. Lily looked over her shoulder at me and said, "Remember this, and remember what I have said." Then she turned and walked back down the pier with my grandmother.

I tried to pull myself out of the water. "Wait!" I cried. "I'm not done yet—there's more I want to say, more I want to know!" But it was too late, they had reached the light and were gone. I started crying again and was floating there, treading water as the whole area grew lighter and the fog lifted—and suddenly I woke up in my bed.

It was so real, and I know it was real because of the way it felt, and because of the people and things that were there. It was still about four in the morning, so I forced myself to go back to sleep. I was hoping I could get back to that pier, and have Lily come talk to me again. It did not happen; my sleep was deep and dreamless after that. When I woke up the next morning, my sadness and feelings of loss and grief were still there, but there was a lightness starting inside me. Because of that dream, somehow things had shifted, and the overwhelming, crushing urge to kill myself and be rid of the endless, unrepairable pain was gone.

There is an interesting point about the dream. When I was pregnant, I felt the baby was a girl, and sometimes had a fantasy about how she would look. In my ideas of her, she looked like my existing three children, just a slightly different version. However, this child in the dream did not look at all as I had pictured her. She looked very much like my boyfriend in features and hair coloring and eye coloring.

As the weeks went by, I remembered the dream over and over again. I tried to make it happen again, but it didn't. However, it was the genesis, even the catalyst of my recovery. As the months went by, I got better. I went to therapy; I worked on healing. When my counselor would ask me, "What do you need to do to get better?" I would think on it for a day or two, and then it felt like an answer would be funneled to me from the other side. Every time I got another answer, I would whisper, "Thank you, Lily."

As I worked on my website for other women trying to heal their lives after an abortion, some nights I would sit down to write at my keyboard, and words, ideas for healing, answers for other women would just pour right out of me. I feel as if some of my writing and healing ideas were channeled directly from Heaven, through my Lily and then to me.

Then Christmas rolled around and I became very sad again. I missed having a little baby to put into a cute red and green sleeper. I looked at my three other children and wondered how they would be sharing Christmas morning with their sister, had she been born. I remembered the Saturday morning in May when I was about six weeks pregnant, lying on the couch fighting the never-ending morning sickness. My five-year-old daughter walked over and laid her hand on my stomach and announced, "My baby sister is in there."

I remember being shocked into speechlessness for a moment, because I had told no one about the pregnancy, and certainly not my children. Her two brothers looked over from their cartoons and said, "No it's not, Mom is not having any more babies!" and I struggled and found my voice again, and weakly agreed with her brothers, and told all three of them, "I am not pregnant, your brothers are right, your sister is not in there." She gazed at me with an incredible look and repeated, "My sister is in there!" then walked away to play. I thought again about that morning, and wanted to ask my daughter about it. But I didn't know where to even start, so I never did.

Christmas passed and New Year's came. Around March I was feeling better, but because of some things my boyfriend had been saying, I started to wonder if it was real, this communication with Lily, or had it just been a regular dream. Was it real? Did I talk to my daughter? Or was it something my brain was making up, to make me feel better? Maybe I was hearing what I wanted to hear? Maybe it was all my imagination?

So I said to the sky, to God, to Lily: "Okay, if this is real, if you really are Lily, and I didn't imagine it all, give me some kind of sign—prove to me that I was not just going through some kind of grief psychosis!" Nothing happened immediately, the sky didn't fall, lightning didn't strike nearby. But I had made my request for proof, for something tangible that would show me clearly whether what I had experienced was real.

The next day I went off to house-sit for two weeks, for a friend of my sister's who was going to Cancun. The woman had a little pet menagerie of birds, cats, a peacock—and one of the six cats was named Lily. Surprisingly enough, the only cat that would come near me, fell instantly in love with me and rubbed herself all over me and slept in bed curled up with me at night for the whole two weeks I was there was Lily! But that's not all.

In the bathroom, there was an old-fashioned picture of a race-horse standing in the winner's circle, wearing the wreath of roses with her jockey. I looked closer; what was the horse's name? "Tac-carro Lily." Interesting, I thought. Two Lilies in a day after I asked for my sign.

The very next day I went in for my normal weekly therapy appointment. I found that their receptionist had suddenly quit, and the new one's name was...Lily. Imagine that! I was starting to see a sign coming. I went home after therapy, and I never watch much commercial TV, but here I was house-sitting, alone and bored, so I turned on a show called "Veronica's Closet" with

Kirstie Allie. There was a special guest character on the show that night, and her name was Lily!

The next morning I went to clean the cat box, with six cats, phew! I couldn't find the outdoor hose. I searched and searched, and finally found it behind a few large pots. In the pots were all these little tags identifying the contents. What bulbs were in these pots? Lilies.

So I go in to work the next day. My boss talks about the new dog she has adopted, and says they decided to name her, you guessed it—Lily. She said the name came to them "out of the blue," that they hadn't ever thought of it before. I didn't share the significance of it all with her, but I was amazed at how many times in just a few days the name Lily showed up! Maybe it was all coincidence, but Lily is not a common name, and it was odd that I suddenly ran into all these occurrences of it right after questioning my faith. I thought it was a clear answer to my request to God and Lily to give me a sign that I could believe in!

And I do believe. I know my Lily is real, I know my communication with her was real, and even now I sometimes feel her around, and get messages from her. This experience has strengthened my belief in a loving afterlife where we continue with our consciousness intact.

20

No Guarantees

o o o o o o o o o o o o o o o o o o o o o o o o o o o o o o o o

I was so sure my visions were premonitions…I was so looking for-
ward to having those glimpses become reality. This really does
seem to mess up my worldview…

—*Kim*

If every vision came true, it would be easy to dismiss the viewpoint of
the psychologist who asked, "How much of this is wishful thinking or
fantasy, combined with a modicum of intuition, and a certain level of
inner processing that provides images and inner dialogue?"

Dreams and premonitions don't always come true. We have experiences that lead us to expect something wonderful—for example, that a
much-wanted child is on the way. Then when years go by and our
hopes fail to materialize, the disappointment is compounded by losing
faith in our intuitions.

People are sometimes baffled by discrepancies between a possible
pre-birth message and the reality that unfolds, such as dreaming
strongly of having a boy but then having a girl. It is an unsettling experience, and I suspect it occurs more often than we realize, because we
tend to forget the predictions that don't pan out. But this is a subject
we need to confront, so as not to give a misleading impression that pre-
birth connections guarantee a certain outcome.

Felicia: Vision of her, birth of him

I have been on an amazing journey in my adult life of self-discovery and recovery. In the last three years I have really begun to listen to my intuition and inner voices and give them credibility. Before that, I thought there was something wrong with me because I saw things or heard voices or felt presences. I still struggle with this, but in my most centered space I know that I am sensitive to information from sources other than what we typically use.

All my life I knew I would have a boy and a girl. When my son was born, it was no surprise. More than two years later, I began sensing a presence of a little girl. She was far away. When I zeroed in on her presence I could visualize outer space. Over several months, she got closer and closer to me, until one morning when I was getting ready for work I saw her behind my right shoulder in the bathroom mirror.

She looked to be toddler age, blond with ringlets in her hair. She looked merry, and had a knowing smile on her face. She was beautiful. I had told my husband that the little girl was probably the soul of our next child waiting to be born. When it got to the point that it almost felt like she was tapping me on the shoulder, we conceived. She disappeared, so my thought was that she was now in my womb.

For seven months we called the baby by her name, and prepared my son for a baby sister. Psychics told us that it was indeed a girl; physical signs in the pregnancy indicated that she was a girl. Seven months of absolute surety went by.

And during those seven months, I was petrified. I have many unresolved issues with my mother, and terrible self-esteem as a result. My fear was that I would pass along my unresolved stuff to this precious little girl. I didn't know if I could be a good mother to a girl. When we had a sonogram to check on the position of the baby, we got the shock of our lives: it was a boy. We were stunned. We quickly set our minds to grieving for the loss of baby Ella, and welcoming the new boy to our family. The last weeks of the pregnancy were spent fervently praying that my second boy would not feel unwanted. His birth was beautiful, as is he. He teaches me every day.

The interesting thing is that my husband and I had decided two children were our limit. No more babies. But neither of us has taken necessary steps to ensure that this decision is final, and now I think I am being visited by this little girl again. My feelings are different this time. I am not so scared about the possibility of having a girl, if we decide to conceive again.

I went through a period of severe self-doubt after learning the baby was a boy. It really rocked my world. It made me wonder if I hadn't been listening to my intuition after all, but was wishful thinking. I have had some supportive woman friends tell me that the little girl may not have been about wanting to be born into physicality, but to help me through some healing. Who knows?

Unfortunately, I have lost touch with Felicia, and don't know whether she went on to have a daughter, more prepared now thanks to the practice run. Her story appeared on my website and drew a response from Kim, who had just experienced a similar shock. Kim explained:

I have had visions of these two, a boy and a girl, for about ten years. In my vision the girl is born first. I have a stronger connection to her, and her presence is more easily sensed. I have had at least two gifted psychics tell me that it would be twins, the girl first, and that the boy may decide not to come at the last minute. My last clear vision was of a little girl spirit zooming me—but then immediately I was handed a boy child clothed in blue. I assumed that meant that I would have the twins.

I was infertile for three years, but now I am seventeen weeks pregnant. Last week I had a sonogram. It is one baby, a boy. No doubt about it. Part of me is devastated, because trusting my intuition is so hard. I am very unsure about all of this now. How could so many have misinterpreted this? I haven't seen or felt my spiritual daughter since I got the news. I am still reeling and numb.

The experiences of Kim and Felicia illustrate a pitfall in pre-birth communication: visionary images don't come with captions to explain them. Our interpretations of them are added on, and often freighted with what we hope they mean. From an outsider's viewpoint, Kim's last vision actually seems to indicate a girl staying in spirit while a boy incarnates, as symbolized by his taking on baby form and blue clothing.

Both Kim and Felicia were assured by psychics that the situation was just as they expected, which made the reality even more shocking. From these and similar stories, it appears that in some cases psychics tune in to ideas in the mind of the mother-to-be. Reflected back by a trusted authority, expectations become certainties. Because of this pattern, I don't pay much attention to input from professional psychics in the stories that are shared with me. I place far more value on personal experience. In my observation, the most reliable information about "who" is on the way will come in one's own dreams. (As we'll see in a later chapter, though, your best bet might be to ask a four-year-old!)

Visions and the F Word

I feel on shaky ground discussing visions, as this category of experience is particularly hard to define. When someone speaks of having a vision, I need details before I can begin to understand just what the word means in this instance.

Some lucky people normally have a pageant of images in full color, unrolling before their mind's eye like a private movie. Others, like me, see nothing behind closed eyes but a dark gray blank. When my daughter was a newborn, however, I did have several vivid mental pictures of "her" as a little girl, like still frames from a dream. They were so unusual for me that I remembered them for a long time, but as she grew older, Rosie did not resemble any of those images. It took years to learn they were not really visions of her future.

I sometimes ask visualizers how they identify a significant vision apart from their usual inner imagery. I'm told the difference is that such images are more vivid, "so clear you could almost touch them," and tend to come unbidden, as strong mental pictures that intrude upon whatever one is thinking and doing. Intensity, clarity, and an element of surprise set these images apart as visions.

I am always curious to know whether the image is perceived inside, or projected in space. Eventually I hope to have more understanding of the various types of visions and be able to offer some guidance as to their reliability, based on experience. For the present, I must say that in general, waking visions seem to be less reliable than dreams, as containers of information that can be verified in time.

But even dreams—even a series of dreams—can lead to disillusionment. A typical disappointment is the promised birth that never happens. There may be dreams, visions, inner messages all pointing to the same outcome, and it can still fail to come true. What went wrong?

If we ignore the possibility of fantasy, we would be denying one of the most wonderful things about our minds: their ability to create virtual reality. We can create these experiences. Anyone who has experienced an altered state (including dreams) recognizes the mind's inventive power. And so, to be honest with ourselves, we have to acknowledge that we may sometimes unknowingly generate a fantasy and invest it with our hope and faith, even cling to it for some kind of security in this insecure world.

Closing Windows and Changing Paths

If some shocks and no-shows are the result of deluding ourselves, this is only part of the story. Even the most definite soul communication still may not "come true" according to our expectations, and so I believe all communications are best received with an open-minded, wait-and-see attitude. There are several possible reasons for the uncertainty.

We've seen evidence of free choice on the part of incarnating souls. This freedom must include the option of reversing a decision. A soul may visit potential parents and make its presence felt, and yet not be committed to entering that family. How long does the unborn soul

hold its option of changing course? Debra York tells a thought-provoking story:

> In an international conference of rebirthers in Hawaii, I remem-
> bered my conception and birth from an out-of-body perspective. I
> remember that after being in labor for three days with no assistance
> from the doctor, when my mother was dying and the fetus was
> already dead, they rushed the mother into the delivery room, jerked
> out the dead fetus and began trying to save the mother. I watched
> this all from the ceiling, remembering having made the decision
> that I would not take a breath until I knew that my mother would
> live because I knew I would not survive this lifetime without her
> love. When I knew she would live, I took my first breath while the
> doctor did mouth to mouth resuscitation. He had tried everything
> else to no avail.

Another possible reason for disappointment has to do with time
frames. When parents-to-be experience a persistent visitor, there is
sometimes the suggestion of a time limit. The window of opportunity
can close. Patricia, for example, was fearful of becoming pregnant
although she had powerful dreams of a little boy for over a year. While
wide awake one day, she finally heard a clear message that this was her
last chance to bear this child, as he had to move on. David Brunner's
story of pre-birth communication was told in Chapter Three. One of
the two children who visited him was not born. David says: "As for
Amy not incarnating, I have often asked this and always get the same
answer, which is that it was too late. My wife and I had separated a
couple times and gotten back together, so the time for her to come into
the earth had been missed."

Communication problems and misinterpretation may account for
some of the surprises. It must not be easy for the unborn soul to convey
a clear message. Information that we receive in a dream, for example,
can undergo changes on its way to conscious awareness. At deeper levels, our knowledge may be more accurate.

An intriguing experiment[1] with pregnant women demonstrates the clarity of unconscious knowledge. Using a hypnotic technique known as ideomotor signaling, twenty-five out of twenty-six women correctly identified the sex of their baby before it was determined by ultrasound. In the one case that was thought to be incorrect according to the sonogram results, it was discovered at the baby's birth that the finger signal was right—it was the sonogram reading that missed! In hypnosis, these women were able to access their subconscious knowledge. If they had been asked to guess in ordinary waking consciousness, their answers would probably have been much less accurate.

After all our questions and efforts to explain confusing experiences, sometimes we are left with mystery. Even repeated and highly specific dreams can be inconclusive. More puzzling still, we can have a mixture of both: pre-birth communications that prove accurate, and others that leave us mystified, perhaps never to know what they really mean.

Janet: The Twin Daughters Mystery

I had a year's worth of communication about having twins. It involved many dreams and synchronicities—so many amazing, inexplicable things that the only conclusion I could draw was that I was being prepared to have twin girls. This was confirmed over and over again.

Here's one example of the unusual things that were happening. Two months after the first twins dreams, I went on a weekend retreat where I internally wrestled with the idea: did I want twins? Was this something I could handle? I strongly sensed I had a choice in the matter. By retreat's end I said to God, to the universe: "Yes, I'm open to this. If these twins have chosen me, I also choose them." The next morning at home, my two-year-old daughter suddenly asked me, "When can I be a big sister?" I told her that as soon as her daddy and I had another baby, she would be the big sister. She said, "Actually, I want two babies. Two girls." She had never before talked of being a big sister, and I hadn't said anything about twins to anyone around me. I had so many other experiences like this, I couldn't record them all.

Six months after the first dream occurred, I became pregnant (announced in dreams before showing on any test), then miscarried that pregnancy at about six weeks (again, forewarned in my dreams days before). The following month, I conceived again. Though an early sonogram did *not* show twins, through the first half of this pregnancy I continued dreaming of twin girls. The dreams became progressively more specific. In the last dream I clearly saw them as older children, knew their names, talked to them, and asked which one was which (they looked identical).

Midway through the pregnancy, another sonogram was scheduled. Ten days before the sonogram, I asked for a dream to tell me clearly what to expect. That night I dreamed that I'd had a baby boy. In the dream I said, "This is not what I expected!" The baby looked at me and said, "We didn't communicate very well at the start."

Part of the dream mentioned the baby's weight. The comment was made, "I was only seven pounds; they didn't think I would make it." Ten days later the sonogram revealed we were indeed having a boy. The dream's comment about weight never made sense to me until our son was born. He came one month early, weighed exactly seven pounds and, as my husband overheard a nurse say, "He almost didn't make it." He spent ten days in Neonatal Intensive Care for various problems, and is now a completely healthy, active nine-month-old.

After the sonogram revealed a boy, I had no more dreams about twins. I have not dreamed of them since, though I do think of them often and wonder if I'll ever know the purpose behind this experience. Because it all was too much, too specific, too unusual to be meaningless.

21

Dakota's Story

As we've seen in the previous chapter, pre-birth communications do not guarantee that events will unfold as we expect. A vision or a dream or even a series of contacts can seem to promise the happy outcome we desire, only to leave us finally wondering if we misunderstood the message, or whether there is some other purpose involved that we never guessed.

Dakota's story is an expression of this mystery. While awaiting the birth of her first child, Kara L.C. Jones related a tender, intimate story of pre-birth communication.

> I moved to Seattle by default. I was hitching a ride this far with my friend Michael who came here to start his career as a chiropractor, and I was eventually heading to San Francisco for grad school. But until then, Seattle seemed like a fine place. I got a job at a local hospital, made friends, and started really liking the Emerald City.
>
> I had worked at the hospital for several months in the Educational Services Department where we did everything from coordinate computer classes to CPR and birthing classes. Every day I walked up a small hill from my bus stop to the hospital, and at the end of each day I walked back down.
>
> One day as I walked to the bus stop after work, I suddenly saw a little girl walking backwards in front of me asking me if I would accept her. I blinked hard and wondered where my head was, as there really was no physical girl walking in front of me! Then I looked to the left and there appeared a man walking with me and asking me if I could see the girl. As this was not an everyday sort of

occurrence for me, I chose to tell the guy, "Yeah, I see her," try to ignore the whole thing, and convince myself that I was not cracking up.

In the following weeks, I had Michael doing adjustments on me using a chiropractic technique called Network. This technique is very subtle, no cracking bones, and often left me relaxed and dreamy. During one of those adjustments, I was lying face down on the table when I suddenly heard the girl again asking me if I would accept her! I looked up and could see her standing there. And again off to my left, sitting on the table next to me was that man asking if I could see the girl. Needless to say, I was a little freaked out. Michael sensed immediately that something was up and asked me about it. I told him about both incidents. He didn't think I was crazy, and he suggested that the next time it happened, I simply ask the girl who she is.

Meanwhile back at the hospital, I had met lots of people and one man in particular, Hawk. I had noticed his midnight voice and knew he was a wonderful computer teacher, but we both went on about our business without really connecting. One afternoon as he was doing some work on my computer, another co-worker returned a copy of my first manuscript of poetry. When she handed the manuscript to me, I swear some Higher Power took over, shoved me aside, handed my work to Hawk and said, "Please read this." He looked surprised, said it often took him a long time to read things as he is dyslexic, and went on his way.

Hawk returned to my desk first thing the next morning with my manuscript in hand and a cassette tape for me. He told me he had been writing music for twenty years, but he hadn't seen the words to his music till he read my poetry. He had taken the manuscript back to his office and started to do his usual thing, which was to skim several pages at random. But the first poem he read brought him to tears. He thought this one poem must be a fluke, but he opened the book to another poem and another and another. Before he knew it, he had read the whole manuscript several times over.

I was flattered by his compliments and stunned to be honored with the tape of his music. I had my Walkman with me, so I quickly listened to the first song. It was a song obviously written for a special woman in his life. And I found myself jealous. Can you imagine? I was jealous of some woman I didn't know and didn't even know if she was still a part of his life. I was jealous that he had written something so beautiful, and it wasn't for me! How silly, I thought to myself. I put the tape away. When I got on the bus after work I listened to his music again, and I had the haunting feeling that I knew this music—all of it. I think I must have listened to the music on that tape for three days straight.

When Hawk and I met again, we decided to spend more time together and maybe write some songs together. For our first "date," we went to Greenlake Park and sat next to the lake on a bright, sunny morning. I had brought a book of poems by Sharon Olds called *Satan Says*. One of the amazing poems in that collection is called "The Unborn," and I read this poem to Hawk. It's about feeling the presence of the children we could have, and how they are waiting and dozing "in some antechamber." In the last stanza it describes one child standing at the edge of a cliff and reaching out its arms "desperately to me."

I hadn't consciously thought, "Oh, let me read him a poem about having children because I want children with this man." I read several others to him that morning, but it was this poem that brought him to question me—did I ever feel like that, like there is a child waiting for me? Well, no. At that point in my life I was doing different kinds of child care work and teaching and that seemed just fine. I told him so. I told him that I love children, but I loved giving them back to their parents at the end of a day or a class. "Oh," was all he said. I think we both knew that in my heart of hearts, I was lying.

Hawk and I spent more and more time together. And as the weeks passed, my visions of the girl got stronger, and she began to enter my dreamstate at night, too. At times the girl was a woman or a boy, but she always had the same familiar voice asking me to accept. Accept what?! And then in a dream I was reminded to ask the girl who she was. So I took Michael's advice and the dream's advice, and the next time I had a strong vision of her during one of my adjustments, I asked. Thank Goddess that Michael had me in a private room this time, because this was pretty emotional stuff.

The child told me that in all forms—girl, boy, woman, or man—she is called Dakota. She told me she wanted to come into human form with me. And she wanted to know if I was going to accept her. Stunned. Over the course of my next few visions/dreams, I came to discover that this child had picked Hawk to be her father. She wanted to know if *we* were going to accept her.

I had no idea how to tell Hawk all this. My relationship with him felt very new, and was I going to risk it all by telling him that I wanted to have a child with him? He had been married before, and already had two teens from his previous marriage. He would think I was insane. But I was overwhelmed with the urge to tell him. I couldn't find my spoken voice to say it all. So in true twentieth century fashion, I typed it all out, proofed it, rearranged the words several times, and emailed him.

He didn't respond for two weeks. At this point I was not working at Educational Services anymore, but in a different area of the hospital. So I literally did not hear from him for two entire weeks. Let me tell you, I went through the whole drama of "Why am I so stupid?" "How could I really think this man would understand?" and "Okay, fine, it's just over!"

Then one afternoon my phone rings. It's Hawk. He says, "I'm ready to talk now." I was stunned. He had been processing this information in a serious way for two weeks. He was surprised, shocked, and ready to talk. At this point, I told him I didn't want to get married. I wanted to go to San Francisco to grad school. But I also wanted to have this child with him. We agreed to make a commitment to each other for life with or without the official marriage thing. Hawk had serious reservations about my being in San Francisco while pregnant and for Dakota's first year or so of life. But we started trying to get pregnant right away.

I lasted in San Francisco for all of about a minute. It was all wrong. My body went crazy on me once I moved there. I started having massive menstrual bleeding; I had a pap smear showing precancerous cells. I was depressed, and I ached to be with Hawk full time. I left San Francisco, Hawk moved me back home to Seattle, and we moved in together. I began intensive healing with acupuncture, meditation, chiropractic, and allopathic medicine, and we kept trying to get pregnant.

I met a wonderful woman who was an obstetrician at the hospital clinic. She took me as a patient to try and sort out what was happening with my body. Subsequent pap smears now showed no pre-cancerous cells! My menstrual periods got light and irregular. We did all kinds of fertility tests and there were questions as to whether or not I could get pregnant at all. My amazing doctor put me on a couple of rounds of a fertility drug, at a very low dose. Nothing. More disappointing minus signs on lots of pregnancy tests.

After a year of this, it was difficult to stay positive, to believe in my dreams and visions, to not start thinking I was just crazy. Hawk and I decided to celebrate Christmas alone. We decided to focus our celebration of the Winter Solstice and Christmas on abundance instead of thinking about disappointment. He sang and played on his guitar a song he had written for me. Some of the words are:

> "In the wind you will hear
> early in the morning
> a sound so sweet and clear
>
> Listen to the wind and you
> will hear Dakota calling you
> and she's saying
> I Love you Mom and I can't wait till I get home…"

Hope, instead of disappointment, began to seep into my heart and soul again. I could hear Dakota's voice so loud and strong in this song. And on this amazing night, Hawk asked me to marry him, to make it official, to be with him forever no matter what. I could not say no this time. I really wanted to be married to him. I wanted God/dess, family, and friends to know out loud and in public that I was in this forever.

We were married on the Summer Solstice. It was a magical day, and Dakota was there for sure. We had lots of family and friends at the wedding who knew about my communications with Dakota. In fact by this time, Dakota had spoken to my Dad in one of his dreams and, in a vision, to a friend who is a brother to me. We had taken some family to Mount Rainier one day and drove up to Paradise to see the snow glittering in the sun. At the top, we split into groups heading for restrooms. When we girls came out, my sister pointed out that some invisible finger had carved the word

DAKOTA in the snow bank. I was certain Hawk had done that for me. But he was as stunned as I was to see it there. He hadn't written it. Neither had I. Neither had anyone who was with us. We were getting used to these "coincidences."

So at our wedding, many people in attendance knew how much and how long Dakota had been with us. Much of the celebration came in the form of fertility ritual and blessings from friends and family. My sister gave us a Fertility Goddess from Ghana as a wedding gift. Sonja, who was both my friend and the minister who married us, gave us a meditation tape for focusing on manifesting Dakota here to the physical plane.

On our honeymoon, we put the Fertility Goddess in a place of honor in our cabin. We took the meditation tape with us as we drove up to Neah Bay one afternoon. We had listened to it for maybe ten minutes when Hawk asked if we could stop the tape and pull over somewhere to finish. He saw a place to pull off that looked out over a small town and the ocean. We parked in front of a boulder that had been spray painted with graffiti. Right in the middle of the boulder, in huge capital letters in blue and white paint was the word DAKOTA.

We came home from our honeymoon and two weeks later, the smell of coffee began making me sick. Finally I summoned up the courage to try another pregnancy test. I was so afraid it would be negative that I couldn't bear to watch it show the results. I made Hawk come into the bathroom and watch it while I stood behind him so I couldn't see it. He said, "Well, honey, this is the biggest, brightest, red plus sign I've ever seen." Ah! We had actually gotten pregnant on our honeymoon!

Not only did Dakota know that he wanted to come to us, not only had he hand picked us, but he knew that I had to completely surrender to love in order to make our lives work. I know that Dakota brought me to Seattle, to that hospital, to Hawk, to Love. And now we are expecting our baby boy, Dakota, to arrive on March 19, 1999, or thereabouts. We spent the holidays this year truly in awe of the abundance we have been guided to.

Kara and I became friends by correspondence as we awaited Dakota's birth. But the letter that came on his due date was a sad shock.

> I have been out of touch for a few weeks. I was sick for a bit with a cold or flu. Last week I was in bed all day and realized that I hadn't felt Dakota move at all since the night before. We rushed in to see our doctor the following morning and they could find no heartbeat in Dakota. We did a sonogram and could clearly see that his heart had stopped. We lost him.
>
> It has been a devastating week, to say the least, and I'm sorry to tell you this sad news by such impersonal means. It doesn't change a bit of what I wrote about Dakota coming to us. But it does change all the expectations we had, you know?
>
> We did have wonderful news today from our doctor, who said we could try to get pregnant again in as soon as three to six months. While this does not make me miss my son any less, it does give me hope and some glimmer of a future that has some distance away from the overwhelming sadness we've been experiencing this past week. The mornings are the most difficult—it's like waking and remembering everything all over again...it seems quite crazy at times.

Two years after Dakota's stillbirth, Kara talks about grief and about the creative project his presence and loss inspired.

> When our baby died, I thought I would go crazy with grief. My husband and I had all this love and energy that we had planned to focus on our child. We didn't know what to do with it. So we made our "creative baby" called KotaPress.[1] Through this company we have created an outreach to other bereaved parents with our Mrs. Duck Project, we have formed an alliance with the Seattle chapter of MISS (Mothers In Sympathy and Support), and we are continually doing projects like Teddy Bear Drives to keep Dakota's memory alive.

In answer to my questions, Kara told more about their communications with Dakota. I was curious to know whether the visionary contacts continued during the pregnancy, and whether Hawk had his own experiences of the unborn soul that seemed to play such a part in bringing them together.

The visions did not stop when Dakota was conceived. If anything, because I was taking hypnobirthing classes which involved a lot of relaxed meditation, the visions were stronger. I visioned Dakota many times while I was pregnant.

Hawk's clearest contacts with Dakota were when the songs (there are several) came to him. He seemed to feel the music and words were guided by a female hand, and he had a clear identification of Dakota as a girl. For me, the first few visions were of a little girl. After that, though, I began working with a hypnotherapist, and in my visions there and in my dreams Dakota started coming to me as girl or boy or woman or man—but I always knew it was Dakota because the voice had the same musical tone or quality to it. Hawk was quite jolted when our sonogram showed us the "outdoor plumbing" of a boy child!

Have we felt Dakota communicating with us since his death? Yes. Constantly. When I was writing *Mrs. Duck and The Woman* just three weeks after his death, he was definitely there in that willow tree where I sat writing as fast as I could, while a duck sat next to me. Most people think the Mrs. Duck story is so cute and wonderful; what they don't realize is that I literally was sitting next to a duck under a willow tree in the park while these words poured out of my fingertips without my mind really being involved—all in twenty minutes. That story is as it was written that day, except that I changed it to say "child" and "baby" rather than son because I wanted it to be relevant for those who had lost daughters, too.

We still have bad days here when we wonder if running Kota Press is right for us or not. We are struggling to make it in an everyday, financial way, and so we wonder if this really is our Path or are we just extending our grief. And something will always happen.

A Dodge Dakota truck will be parked at random in our parking space outside the house. A woman from Seattle will be visiting an Interfaith Church in the Midwest and mention to the pastor there that she hasn't found any grief support in her home town. That pastor will happen to be someone I just finished emailing with about the Mrs. Duck Project, and a connection is made. I will have a horrid day and think this is pointless, and I want to give it up because nobody cares and no one needs another grief support and no one wants to sponsor this Project anyway. And I'll suddenly get fifty email messages, one right after the other, from families requesting Mrs. Duck support...

Mind you, we are still struggling. I am still having my faith tested. I'm still on the edge every day here, but when these "coincidences" happen, I just can't ignore Dakota's footprints all over it!

Have we come to some sort of insight on "what it's all about"? *Goddess*, I just don't know. I think that we weren't living "authentic lives" before Dakota died. We were in a situation where we worked for a paycheck, we slaved for corporate America, and we were consumers. I was definitely on the high and mighty academic path in terms of my writing career. And although we are struggling now to do simple things like pay rent and make car payments, I think these are struggles we were meant to face and resolve somehow.

I think we were meant to do something authentic, something creative, something that has a healing meaning behind it. I think I was meant to get real with my writing, to see resource rather than the competitive point of view that was fostered in my academic experiences. I think we are living closer to the ground now, we have dirt under our fingernails, we are sober, we are painfully aware of joy and sorrow and something real that we didn't have when we were blissfully, blindfully shopping at BabyMart to have the best crib, the best changing table, the best toys, the best blah blah blah that seemed so important when I was pregnant with Dakota.

The word "Dakota" is a Sioux word meaning friend or ally. I think Dakota came, lived, and died as our friend and ally.

22

Traces of a Plan

It wasn't until she was expecting her third child that Kendra* finally put into words her own pre-birth memories, hoping to find someone who could relate to them. "After burying them for so long," she says, "the details are not very clear any more." But in fact, this was not the first time she tried to talk about her memory of conception:

> I told my mother about it when I was very small but she dismissed it as a dream. I remember someone asking me if I would go to her—to be my mother's daughter because she needed me. I remember agreeing, and there was a blue light and I was above her in her room. She was sleeping next to a man who I knew was not important to me. I was somehow flashed inside of her. I don't know how to describe it well...
>
> For a while I don't remember anything. Then I remember being inside her and it was warm and there was an orange-red glow in front of me. It felt like all time was suspended in there. My mother was happy I was there. The man who had been lying beside her did not want me, but he did not matter. I remember someone else talking to me when I was inside her, maybe God.
>
> My father tried to make her get an abortion, even dragging her to the clinic and hitting her until she passed out, but I know I felt safe. I don't actually remember her being dragged to the clinic, but I remember the stress of not being wanted by him. That was when I was reassured that I was meant to be now, and the abortion wouldn't happen.

I was about two or three when I tried to tell my mother about my memories. I think she could have been more open, but she is grounded in beliefs that would rule out any existence before conception. Even though I learned a lot from her, she always says I should have been the mother, and it did seem that way. She does and says such off-the-wall kid type things, even now at forty-three. I think my being in her life was important and helpful for her. She was heavily on drugs until she found out she was pregnant with me at six weeks; then she stopped everything and turned her life around. She says she learned so much from me; if she needs to understand something she just asks me and I tell her, and it's as if it was meant to be like that.

If there are purposes behind our family combinations, we should be able to detect traces of them somewhere. And we do find such traces, but we need to go beyond stories of pre-birth communication. Memories, whether retained throughout life like Kendra's or discovered in hypnosis, can carry echoes of a conversation guiding the soul on its way to the world. Similarly when people undergo a near-death experience, they sometimes recover the memory of a purpose or a promise made before birth that still remains to be fulfilled:

Pamela: "Oh yeah. I forgot!"

When I was about eight or nine years old, I was swimming in a pond with my family and I drowned. I remember thinking, "Don't you only go down three times? One. Two. Three. This is four times!" Then I was lying on the bottom of the pond thinking, "Hey, I don't need to breathe. This is neat!" I could see black, warm darkness, then a bright light. I thought, "The sun looks so big and bright down here. I could stay here forever."

I felt a large hand (I thought of it as God) lift me to the surface. The colors were so bright, brighter than any I had ever seen. I felt I could see forever. The hand slowly turned me around. I could see my mother surrounded by my father and cousins and I could feel what they were feeling. Everyone thought something was wrong with my mother. She was scared—she could not talk. She was thinking her Pammy was drowning. Then a voice told me, "She needs you." I remember that my response was, "Oh, yeah. I forgot." I was dropped back into my body and I began to choke and struggle to live.

It seemed I had a prior obligation to the woman who was my mother. I do not know if this was from a past life or a pre-life contract, but even as a young child I knew I had a purpose for my life. I did not know that my mother was to die four years later after a long illness.

"From a past life or a pre-life…" Hints of other lifetimes, or reincarnation, are scattered throughout stories of soul memory and pre-birth communication. There is abundant evidence for some form of rebirth, particularly in the research of Dr. Ian Stevenson, though I suspect that "the way it works" may be different from the ways we are able to imagine it in our limited three-dimensional state. Terms like re-incarnation and pre-existence imply a time sequence, but time may be the ultimate red herring on our path to understanding.

People who have pre-birth memories don't invariably remember other lifetimes. Some do; others do not. Monica, for example, remembers being with her grandmother in a pre-existence, but does not believe in reincarnation because she recalls specifically knowing that she had never yet been born but existed as spirit.

Artist and child advocate Deborah Barr states another point of view: "In pre-birth communication, love and bonding are very important, but I believe that it is the shared past life experiences which determine the relationship with the child. I believe that our souls are like magnets and 'like attracts like.' I also believe we have agreements to help another soul through a lifetime, to be the strong one. My son Daniel and I have such an agreement." A spontaneous recall provided Deborah with the key to this soul pact:

Deborah: "If only I was Mom"

My first past life memory with Daniel was when he was eight months old. I was lying in bed cradling him in my arms. My other two children were asleep. He had been fussing and had just fallen asleep too. It was a warm fall evening, the sun was down and my husband was still at work.

I closed my eyes and within a few seconds was viewing a movie—I don't know what else to call it. It was as if I was looking at a movie screen only I was in the movie. Suddenly I was inside a covered wagon. I could hear the rain hitting hard against the tarp, and the pots and pans hitting the side of the railing. I could hear the horse's hooves, and the wheels grinding over the ground.

I was a boy of about ten years old and my sister lay before me in the back of the wagon, dying. She was five, blond with blue eyes, very petite and frail. I began sobbing and crying. The sorrow I felt cannot be described.

I knew our mother had died, and that my father was in the front of the wagon driving the horses and could not stop for we would be lost behind the rest of the wagon train. My sister was so weak and sick; she had pneumonia. I could do nothing to help her. I kept telling her, "If only you were a boy like me you would have been stronger. If only I was Mom, I could stop the sickness." I looked deeply into her eyes right before she died.

I left the altered state of consciousness and I was in my room again, holding my baby. I realized as I cried that I was holding my little sister. I had come back as her mother, and she had come back as a boy.

I had several regressions after this, and many times remembered the boy of ten whose name was Alexander, though his sister and family called him "Butch." I would think of my sister often and in my regressions would even see "remembering her" after her death. When Daniel was five, he volunteered validation of my experiences. I had never talked to him about this life together and my past life recalls; I felt it wasn't right to impose my beliefs on him.

I was in the kitchen, cooking dinner and he was being a boy, obnoxious as usual. I was getting after him to behave when he said, "Well, you used to lock me in the tool shed." I turned around and

said, "You used to get me in trouble." I stopped dead in my tracks.
I had to think about what I had just said; it was not a conscious
statement. We didn't have a tool shed. I never locked my son in
any room, not even his. And how in the world could he get me in
trouble? I asked him casually, "When was this, Daniel?" His reply
was, "When you were my brother." I said, "Did I do that?" He
said, "Yeah, when I was a girl."

I calmly thought about his statement. Daniel would never admit
to being a girl, he was all boy! I asked him my name; he said, "You
were Butch." Then he added, "My name was Alicia." Then he told
me not to tell anyone; he didn't want his friends to know. He took
off running out of the room, playing as usual.

He seemed to move in and out of an altered state of consciousness with ease; I admire that in children. Daniel seemed to remember what I knew from regressions and visions. He is a beautiful,
sweet boy with a heart of gold, but school is very hard for him. It's
not that he's not smart. I know it's just that he has had very few
lives where he had an education. Either he didn't live long enough,
there was no schooling for that culture, or he was a girl and girls
were not educated. I have agreed to protect him and hold his hand
through this lifetime, assuring his education, health, and happiness.
I am his rock...his foundation.

Deborah's amazing story shows the enactment of wishes made in
the former life: that "Butch" could be the mother, that the frail girl
would be a sturdy boy, and that Butch as Deborah would be able to
protect her/him. These ardent wishes, spoken to the dying child and
held by both brother and sister, seem to have guided their rebirth in a
new relationship. It is a fascinating glimpse of how our desires may set
the pattern of our soul's next act.

Instead of grand missions, we've found traces of a rather humble
and practical purpose: to help another soul on life's difficult road. Will
we see our children differently, if we realize that among other purposes
they may be here to help us?

The next story brings us back to a pre-birth communication experience. Here the evident link from life to life is the desire to pick up rela-

tionships that were interrupted, and to continue them in a new and more favorable context.

Rick: Together again…in a way it was meant to be

Twenty-one years before the birth of my first granddaughter, I was a young man serving in Vietnam and engaged to be married. Sadly, my fiancé killed herself in June of 1969. From that day on, I dreamed about her off and on until 1994.

When my daughter was going to have a baby, I only knew that it was a little girl. The day before she gave birth I had a dream. I was on a bus, and the girl I had dreamed about for the last twenty years was once again sitting beside me. She told me it was time for her to come back into my life. We talked and talked what seemed like forever, about how we can share something very special, a chance to be with one another again in a way it was meant to be.

My granddaughter and I have a very strong bond, one that I even find hard to accept at times. Even my wife Lori agrees that this is the girl I was going to marry so long ago. The kicker is—Lori was her best friend.

For a short time when she was between two and three years old she said and did things that made my wife and me look at each other, as if she were saying things to us from the past. When she was about three or four, she saw some pictures taken of Lori and me in Hawaii. No one had told her that the pictures were of Hawaii, but she took one look at them and said, "That's Hawaii and I've been there." She only mentioned this the first time she saw them and never again, but we knew what she meant. I had met my fiancé in Hawaii in 1969 when I was stationed in Vietnam.

My fiancé was a dancer, and my granddaughter wanted to dance right away. She has been in dance class for two years and can't wait to go each week. She is extra happy to be around us, much more so than the other grandchildren.

I like to think this story is true, but you know it may just be all in my mind and could be a way to deal with something that happened so long ago. I'm not sure; but I still feel this connection is something special and has been for many lives. I'm not going to tell her of my dream or anything about what we think may be true. Just to have her back in our life as our granddaughter is more than a blessing.

Lori adds: "When my husband told me of his dream about our granddaughter, I was taken aback. However, the instant I saw her and held her I knew there was something extra special about her. There is a connection beyond just the love of a grandparent. She has just turned six and that bond seems to get stronger. I do believe there is something after death, and the bond I had with my girlfriend is now being continued through my granddaughter."

Sometimes I forget that it's not all about parents. Our children are not here just for us, but for each other and who knows what relationships that beacon most brightly to them. In the next two chapters, we will explore one of the most tender and heartening patterns to emerge from pre-birth communication stories: the Grandparent Link.

23

The Grandparent Link

o o o o o o o o o o o o o o o o o o o o o o o o o o o o o

We think the ancestors are behind us, but they are actually those who go before us. They are a vanguard, a spirit wave that pulls us along.

—Joan Halifax, *The Fruitful Darkness*

During my pregnancies, I felt especially close to my Italian grandparents, who had passed away many years before. I remembered them more clearly than usual and I felt the atmosphere of their home all around me, like a waking dream enfolding me in warmth. I pondered whether they might be returning as my children. Was this the reason for their presence in my thoughts, or did I simply crave the memory of their kindness, the way you do crave things in pregnancy?

Or perhaps my grandparents were near, as companions to the souls coming to be born in our family. In previous chapters, we've seen a grandmother hand in hand with Jilly's aborted child (Chapter Nineteen) and a grandfather taking care of Tara's daughter awaiting birth (Chapter Ten). The connection between grandparents and unborn souls has come up often enough to change my ideas about family.

My mother often tried to interest me in our family tree, but I was a spiritual snob and maintained that my soul's lineage had nothing to do with our line of ancestors. My view was too limited; stories of pre-birth communication have shown me that family bonds are important and enduring. The power of love from generation to generation may be greater than we guessed. For some of us at least, the soul's history and family history are woven together. Monica's story illustrates this connection in the pre-birth world.

Monica: On Grandmother's lap

Ever since I was about three years old, I've been telling my mom about my grandmother. I used to pass pictures of her in the house and tell my mom how much I missed sitting on her lap. Mom would get upset and tell me that I never sat on my grandmother's lap because she died six years before I was born. She was certain I was getting the picture mixed up with someone I'd met somewhere else. And I was certain I was not.

As I grew older, instead of doubting, I became more and more convinced I really had a memory and was not at all confused. There was just too much detail. I actually remember sitting on my grandmother's lap in a rocking chair. It was in a large, white room. There were no walls that I could see, but I was aware that the boundary was there. I also remember knowing I was not an adult. I was what I considered a "baby spirit." I was not yet born, I had never been born yet but still I existed in heaven.

I know my grandmother was telling me all about my life and some of the important decisions I was going to have to make. She was trying to give me some guidance to make my life a little easier. It worked. I have been aware from a very young age that I seemed to have wisdom beyond my years when it came to making certain decisions. I was aware that I seemed to be different in my philosophy, almost too adult for a child, yet it was second nature to me.

As I grew older I began having dreams. From the very beginning I knew these were not ordinary dreams; they were dreams about the future. They always take place in the same "white" room, and they always come true. It doesn't seem strange to me any more to dream the future. I just take them as a gift from God. I've made some very important, life altering decisions based on these dreams, and I've always made the right choice.

Grandparents in spirit take an interest in the new arrivals to their family, and form various kinds of relationship with them. They appear as guides, as guardians, and as messengers announcing a pregnancy. Mothers often speak of feeling the presence of grandparents and other ancestors at the birth of a child, as if the generations are gathering in celebration and support. From the Philippines comes the story of a great-grandmother's visit to the new baby:

Rhodora: The woman in the lamplight

When I was a baby only a little over a month old, my mother had me on the bed beside her so she could breastfeed easily. She woke up in the middle of the night to go to the bathroom, and when she came back she saw, in the light of a kerosene lamp, a woman bending over me as if to kiss me. She screamed, and the woman hesitated and slowly disappeared.

My father woke up and asked her what happened. Mother described the visitor as a short, very fair older lady wearing a long skirt and a blouse with three-quarter sleeves, the costume of fifteen to twenty years before. My father was amazed because the description was perfect for his deceased grandmother, whose favorite grandson he was. He said she was short and very fair and had a singing voice like an angel's.

You can imagine how this story made me feel. It underscored the ties between generations and made me feel loved and special. So sometimes, when I feel like singing (something I do only for my own amusement), I think of that great-grandmother and send her my love, wherever she is.

Grandparents Announce the New Arrival

Sometimes a deceased grandparent brings the news of a baby on the way, or reveals whether the child is a boy or girl. Angela Di Meglio's mother had already given birth to three boys and felt sure she was carrying another son. But then her mother-in-law appeared in a dream and announced, "You're going to have a beautiful baby girl." Says

Angela, "She told no one of this dream until I was born, at which point she gave me the name of the grandmother who had visited her."

In visitations from grandparents, they often appear in a younger form, as they looked many years before their old age. I love this detail and consider it a mark of psychological truth. Now that age is changing my looks, I realize (despite much propaganda about the beauty of age) that my younger face was a more faithful representation of "me." In the next announcing dream, the visitor's youthful appearance (unknown to the dreamer) provided evidence of her identity.

W. Davis: "This is your daughter"

My grandmother passed away when I was in the sixth grade. It affected me, but not as it would if it were to happen today. At that age you forget things.

At fourteen I was told I would never be able to have a child, that the endometriosis had returned too many times despite two surgeries and drug-induced menopause. About a year after high school, I ran into a high school acquaintance I never would have been interested in before. He was great; we talked and laughed, he let me be me and inspired me to follow my own dreams. We fell in love and I knew he wanted to ask the question. The fact of no children lay in the back of my mind. When the subject finally did come up, his response was that it was fine, we'd adopt. So we planned the big ceremony, bought the dress and had it all arranged. It was his idea to make an appointment to see a fertility specialist just to see what our chances were. Laughing, I took him up on it and with complete skepticism made the appointment.

About a week after setting the appointment I was not feeling well. I went to bed early that night and I will never forget what followed.

I was dreaming, no doubt about that. There was a woman, dressed in white as if she was in a flowing gown. We were in a cloudy, foggy place, almost as though we were standing on clouds. I believe in God but I am not religious, so I was surprised to be in the presence of such an angelic figure. The figure was quite a ways away and she seemed to slowly creep forward. As she came forward

I kept repeating, "Hello? Hello, can I help you?" Suddenly she was face to face with me. She had beautiful brown hair, smooth silky skin, and eyes that could light up any room.

The woman was holding something in a blanket and as I looked down she raised my head by lifting my chin. She said, "I can only show you this for a second, my love, just a second." She then uncovered a beautiful sleeping baby. I looked right at her and asked, "What does this mean? Who is that?" As she covered the baby up again she said, "This is your daughter, my love, your daughter." I wanted to hold and touch the baby and when I asked to I was told, "Not yet, my love. You must be patient." When I awoke next morning I was so calm, so happy, and had a peaceful feeling all day long.

As the appointment with the fertility specialist grew nearer, my mother and I had many heart to heart talks about disappointment and optimism. One day the dream came up and I began telling her about it. She was sitting across the table drinking her coffee and immediately she started to cry. She got up, walked to the bedroom and returned with a small photograph. The woman in that picture was the woman with my baby. She was twenty-five years old, beautiful, vibrant, my grandmother. I had never seen this picture, let alone ever knew what my grandmother's hair color had been, before the beautiful gray that I remembered.

Two days after that discussion with my mother I felt ill while having dinner at a local restaurant. It was just upset stomach so I excused myself from the table and went to the bathroom. After washing my face with cold water I returned to the table, to my mother with a huge smile on her face: "You're pregnant." I was shocked to hear that from my mom. "We're going to get a test," she said. I told her no way, why waste my money. She said, "Fine, I'll buy it. If it comes back positive, you buy the dinner, negative I will." So on the way home we stopped and got a test. We returned to her house and I took the test. Both of us were sitting on the floor in the bathroom to wait out the three minutes. Sure enough, it was positive.

During my sixth month we were pleased to discover through a sonogram that we were having a girl. Now I truly believe my daughter was sent to me for a purpose. I cannot tell you she looks like the baby in my dream because I can't remember that baby exactly. But I do believe I had a glimpse of what we were going to be blessed with in life.

Grandparents as Guides and Guardians

Grandparents in spirit sometimes appear as guides, accompanying the unborn soul, or like guardian angels offering help. The following stories are especially moving, as they show how love and concern endure down through generations. Here, grandparents advise and comfort young parents in trouble.

Kasey Bowling: The Lady in Mauve

Ever since I was a little girl I have had dreams of a blond Lady. She was there whenever I thought of her. When I was about five she came to me and told me she would only be there when I needed her most. Since then I have only had four dreams of her; two were when she told me that my grandfathers had passed on and that they were safe and with her, and the third one is the subject of this story!

When I was twenty I got engaged and pregnant. My fiancé was nineteen and a Marine in Jacksonville, North Carolina. At first we were ecstatic but that ended when we told our parents, who promptly informed us we were not ready for this responsibility and threatened to disown us if we had this baby. This was coming from both our families! Being young and easily persuaded, we decided together that the most responsible decision would be to terminate this pregnancy.

When I was in the clinic and half way through the procedure I had a morality wake-up scream! I asked the doctors if it was too late to stop, if I could still have the baby if they stopped. They told me it was too late and the baby was already gone. I cried all that day; I felt I was a murderer and no one could change my mind. In many ways I still feel this way.

That night after I had gone to bed I woke up to the feeling that someone was in the room with me. I opened my eyes to see the blond Lady dressed in mauve silk and holding a baby wrapped in the same material. She told me that the baby was all right and she was with her and both of my grandfathers and they would take care of her and love her till I would join them! I asked if I could see the baby's face (still my biggest curiosity to this day). The Lady told me that in the end there would be all the time in the world to know all about her, but now she would be looking after me and not vice versa as it would have been if she was born.

I named the baby Rheanna Jane. She is my littlest guardian angel and I can feel her around me at all times every day.

When I got back to California I had a heart to heart talk with my mother and told her about the blond Lady. She asked me to describe her and when I did, my mother turned white as a ghost. She said she knew this woman, she had seen pictures of her. Her name was Giovanna Palarmo and she was my great-grandmother. She had died in childbirth in her late twenties almost eighty years ago!

About a year later, around the anniversary, I had another dream about Giovanna. I was very depressed and lonely. She came to me and told me to stop dwelling on the past and stop crying. She said that Rheanna loves me and understands my choices, and that I would have plenty of time to be a mother because I was going to have a little boy when I am twenty-five and twins when I am twenty-eight. Being twenty-two now, I am enjoying my childless years knowing in the future I have my work cut out for me. Also I have two nieces and two nephews who keep their auntie quite busy!

Jenn Cramer: Hannah's guardian angel

As a youngster, I had a tremendous relationship with my great-grandmother, Mum Mum. She was both my teacher and my favorite playmate. My Mum Mum died when I was thirteen. I was saddened with her parting, but I knew some day I would see her again.

In my senior year of college, I found out my fiancé and I were expecting. I was terrified. I did not think I was prepared at all! When I was nine weeks pregnant, my Mum Mum was at the foot of my bed while I was up reading one evening. She sat down on the edge of the bed and told me I was ready, all I had to do was listen to my heart in deciding what to do, how to care for myself during the pregnancy, caring for the baby afterwards, and so on. Then she left. I had so much to ask her about what to do that I really took no heed of her advice, and listened to others instead of myself.

In my seventh month, I was sleeping on my grandparents' porch swing when she came back into my life again. I was finally starting to love the idea of being a mother, and was actively talking and reading to my baby. However, I had made a mistake in assuming I was going to have a little boy—hoping actually, because I was, and still am, a true tomboy. Mum Mum showed up on that back porch and up the steps behind her walked this beautiful blond-haired, blue-eyed child. I couldn't say anything, and the little one smiled at me and said, "I hope you'll love me as much as I love you." I could do nothing but smile and say, "Of course, Hannah," and that name just popped out of nowhere.

Needless to say, I had a baby girl, blond and blue-eyed, named Hannah, the most ladylike child you've ever seen. My great-grand-mother was not done yet, though. When Hannah was three weeks old, she visited to tell me Hannah's eyesight was in danger and to get her to a doctor right away. (Hannah had been born with the use of forceps, and her eye was bruised.) The next day I made an appointment for her to see her eye doctor, and she had conjunctivi-tis. With her previous condition, she might have gone blind in that eye if we hadn't "noticed" it as soon as we did. I strongly believe Hannah has a true guardian angel.

Grandparents' Gifts

I don't know of anything more moving and comforting than the many ways grandparents in spirit connect with us. They manifest themselves after death, offering reassurance; they are encountered in near-death experiences, guide unborn souls to the world, act as guard-ian angels, and may even return into the family as new babies. Jenn Cramer, whose "Mum Mum" accompanied her little girl, experienced another grandparent connection. She relates:

When I was fourteen, my grandfather died in a car accident while my immediate family and I were on vacation. At approximately the time of his accident, my parents, my brother and I had just settled into our camper to go to sleep. I was not yet asleep. My grandfather appeared before me and told me, "I'm going to have to leave you for a while, but I'll keep popping in to check on you. If you ever need me, listen to the wind." (I do not know why he said that, but it works. Whenever I visit his gravesite, I can hear his voice in the wind.) After he said this, he faded away, and I felt very peaceful...

Stories like this are thrilling, and yet it is only one's personal experience that can satisfy the desire to know whether we exist after death. For me, the convincing contact happened at age thirteen, when I was jolted from the edge of sleep one morning by a tangible, audible, shocking kiss on my cheek. More telling than the event itself was my body's reaction. After a few seconds of paralyzed stillness, I felt my heart slow and pound with scary, shuddering force. My conscious mind didn't know what had happened, but my body knew it had been touched by a powerful, unearthly energy. Half an hour later, we received news that my grandmother had died the day before, halfway around the world. Then it fell into place; I knew what I had felt.

Besides evidence of life beyond death, I find joy in the surrounding details. Grandmother died in advanced old age, blind and deaf, disoriented since a recent fall from bed and no longer able to recognize her beloved daughters who cared for her around the clock. Yet within a day of passing from the body, her "unborn soul" found me in a distant country and delivered an awesome bolt of energy.

Still, this experience is convincing only for me. Husband and son have heard me tell it, but neither one thinks life after death is likely. I don't mind, though. Of the three of us, I'm the only one who has a chance of saying "I told you so!"

24

Grandparents Returning?

One day when my daughter was about six, she flopped down on the bed, fixed me with her clear gaze and asked an unexpected question: "Is this my first life or my second life?" Before I could come up with an answer, she provided her own: "It's my second life—I was your grandmother last time!"

Evidence of reincarnation? Maybe…but during her early years I was gathering accounts of unusual experiences around childbirth; she may have heard me commenting on the connection between grandparents and new babies that cropped up so often in the stories. Still, those same stories tell me that her announcement could well be true.

While researching children's past life memories, Carol Bowman discovered a common pattern of rebirth into the same family. In *Return From Heaven*, she documents cases of children who display the memories and mannerisms of deceased relatives, including grandparents and great-grandparents.

Many families have their own hand-me-down anecdotes, bits of lore linking personalities from different generations. Angela Di Meglio's family cherishes a story of when Angela was a toddler and her grandmother was babysitting her. In Angela's words, "Grandmother yelled at me for being stubborn and I said in reply with an unusually clear tone, 'When I was the mommy and you were the little girl, did I talk to you like that, Margie?' and my grandmother exclaimed, 'Oh, God, Mom's come back to haunt me!'"

A funny family story—but the implications are profound.

If reincarnation is a reality, and if the soul has some choice about its new parents, then a loving connection with a grandchild could be a natural pathway back to the world. Perhaps we can even plan ahead now to return in a future generation of our family. The philosopher (and heavy drinker) Alan Watts may have done exactly that, according to his daughter Joan. Near the end of Watts's life, Joan told him of her unfulfilled desire to have another child.

> "After I'm dead," Watts told her, "I'm coming back as your child. Next time round I'm going to be a beautiful red-haired woman." He had written of the "completely rational" belief in reincarnation that he held. He thought that the energy that had made him in the first place was bound to do it again in some other form. "After I die I will again awake as a baby."
>
> Joan was not sure how lighthearted he was being in his promise to return as her child, but not long after his death she did conceive and eventually gave birth to a very pretty red-haired daughter, Laura, whose character sometimes reminded Joan of her father. Once, when Laura was a tiny girl, she and Joan visited a friend's house, and Laura went to the cupboard where the liquor was kept, pushed a number of bottles out of the way, reached in, and removed a bottle of vodka from the back of the cupboard. Joan laughs as she tells this story, neither quite believing nor disbelieving her father's promise.

A friend and I were chatting about the uncanny wisdom of our little girls. Roberta confided that she believes her daughter Hilary may be her grandmother reborn. "There is a strong physical resemblance between Hilary and my mother's mother," she says. "Of course that may be genetics, but it extends to facial expressions that make my Mom say, 'Oh God, that was just like my mother!'"

Hilary has habits and personality traits that were typical of her great-grandmother, such as a fondness for wearing old-fashioned kerchiefs on her head and a penchant for practical jokes. "At the age of two," Roberta recalls, "she always pretended to be mixing ingredients and baking—and I'm not a baker but Grandma was—and she would say 'shugah' with what sounded like Grandma's New York accent." The most startling incident took place when Hilary was only about eighteen months old. While Roberta was putting her to bed one night, Hilary looked up and announced, "I'm the Grandma, you're the child!" Roberta reflects, "My grandmother died when I was six, and all through my life I wished that I had known her."

From Australia, Miradija's story is like a mystery, with subtle clues mounting up over time and leading her to make a tentative identification of grandparents reborn among her children.

Miradija: Enduring Romance

My grandmother died when I was thirteen years old, and I was devastated. I had always expected her to be there to see my children grow up. When I was nineteen and pregnant with my first child, I seemed to grieve all over again for my grandmother. The night my son Tyler was born, when they placed him into my arms, I started crying. My husband asked if I was crying because my mother had missed the birth. I told him I was crying because I missed my grandma, and I wished she were here to see my son.

Time passed, and when Tyler was three, I was pregnant with my third child. After two boys, I was hoping for a girl. When I was about twelve weeks pregnant and hadn't yet told my boys we were having another baby, Tyler ran past me and patted my stomach, and said, "Ha ha, I touched your baby." My mother's jaw and mine both dropped!

I couldn't work out what I'd call the new baby, and I joked to someone that I wished babies came with name tags. My friend told me that when I went to bed I should ask my spirit guide what name my child had chosen for itself. So that night I did just that. When I woke up, I had the name "Eva" on my lips, which was my grandmother's name. Two cousins had already been named Eva, so I didn't want to upset anyone, and told no one of the name that had come to me. A few weeks later, my mother asked me very quietly if

I had thought of the name Eva. I told her then what had happened, and she said I really should name her that. I disagreed. I asked Tyler what we should name the baby, and he immediately said, "Karen" which was my mother's name. We laughed, not thinking anything of it.

Meanwhile, I was having dreams of a beautiful baby girl with black wavy hair and greenish eyes, and my mother had told me that my grandmother was a baby with black wavy hair, and she had greenish eyes. (My boys both were blond and blue eyed.)

I gave birth to my daughter, and as soon as my mother held her, she said, "Oh, Eva." I kind of cringed, because I still hadn't decided on a name. But when she was placed into my arms, I had a warm sensation and I began to cry, and said, "She's definitely Eva." She had black wavy hair, and her eyes were not blue like my boys' eyes.

Soon my sister brought my sons to the hospital to see their new sister. My older son, Tyler, wouldn't leave her. When the nurses were giving her a bath and her shots, he told me to leave him there with his sister and the nurses. So I did. That afternoon, when my mother returned to the hospital she was laughing and holding a pink rose. She said, "I think this rose was meant for you," and told me how her rosebush in the back garden, which had never flowered, had produced one pink rose that morning.

We got home from the hospital and Tyler hardly left Eva's side. When she cried, he would run into her room, hold her hand and sing to her, and instantly she would stop crying.

Twelve months passed, and on Eva's first birthday the rosebush produced another pink rose. It was then that we thought of a connection, and I asked my mother to keep the rose for me.

Then Tyler started saying very strange things. He asked me, "Remember when I was your grandpa?" I told him he couldn't have been my grandpa, because he was my son, and my grandpa had died before I was born. Then he said, "I remember when my grandma was my baby." I stared at him, and reminded him that it was impossible, because he was my son. He then repeated, "No, Grandma was *my* baby." (My mother was the youngest of six children in her family.) I was shocked, and then just said to him, "Oh, okay then." I was too shocked to say any more.

I told my mother what Tyler had said and she began to cry, and told me how she had felt a special bond with Tyler and Eva. Then we pulled out the photo album, and the resemblance between my son and my grandfather was uncanny! My second son has full pouty lips, as does my daughter, but Tyler has thin lips. My grandfather had lips exactly the same; his eyes were the same, his hair was the same, his face shape—everything. This brought goosebumps to both of us.

My grandmother's full name was Eva Mary. One day my husband was talking to our sons and asking if they knew their middle names. Tyler promptly started rattling off everyone's full names, but when he got to Eva (her full name is Eva Anne Dawn), he said, "And Eva's is Eva Mary." Our jaws dropped, as no one had ever actually mentioned my grandmother's middle name before. So I said, "No, Tyler, Eva's middle name isn't Mary; think again." Then he said, "Oh that's right, it's Eva Mary Dawn." I had to correct him, and I told him Eva's whole name was Eva Anne Dawn. He looked a little confused at first, then he just added, "Oh, that's right."

To this day, at five and two years old, Tyler and Eva are as close as ever. I don't doubt they have been together in a former life. He takes care of her from the moment she wakes up, running around doing things for her. The first thing he does when he comes home from school is give her hugs and kisses.

He had a school play about two months ago, and we were in the audience watching. We almost had to restrain her from running up on the stage. She was calling to him all the way through, and he was smiling and giving her cheeky grins. Once their play had finished, we allowed Eva to run up to him, and he grabbed her in a bear hug and spun her around. It was so beautiful. Then he chased her around for five minutes until we had to leave. Leaving was hard; she started crying for him, and he started crying too. Even his teacher came up to me and commented on how close they looked.

Tyler has made many other comments. At first I was just brushing them off, thinking nothing of them, but then they became so I couldn't deny what he was saying any longer.

The sequel to this tender story came two years later, when Eva at four and a half made a remarkable comment to her mother. Miradija relates:

> We were sitting in my car and Eva said to me, "When you were a little girl, I was your Gjushi." (She calls my mother this; it means Grandmother in Albanian.) She went on, "You never cried for me when you were little."
> I said, "Really? Why didn't I cry?"
> "Because you love me."
> I straightaway told my mother this, and she told me that when she went shopping and left me with my grandmother, when she returned my grandmother would say, "She never cried for me, she's a good girl." I must admit, I'm quite chuffed!

Miradija mentions the resemblance between her grandfather and her son Tyler. In apparent cases of reincarnation, the physical similarities can go beyond features. Some children have birthmarks that mimic wounds from a former life. (Recall Sobonfu Somé's description of a mark placed upon miscarried or stillborn babies, to help identify them in a new birth.) Even more mystifying, some babies are born with complications or health problems echoing the circumstances of a previous death.

Leslie had many vivid dreams about her unborn baby during her second pregnancy. In one dream, she saw herself with a baby boy. Then she heard a man's voice saying, "Remember, when you are taking care of me, that you already know who I am." A few days before the birth, she made a request while going to sleep: "If I already know who you are, who are you?" To continue in her own words:

"I dreamed of my grandfather looking at me and laughingly saying, 'You and I have a lot in common.' Well, that was more excitement than I could stand, as nothing seemed to have devastated me more in life than the death of my grandfather when I was thirteen. I had always secretly hoped and felt that someday my child would be my grandfather and that the gap that had been made with his passing would be made whole again."

Leslie's son was born within a day or two of the anniversary of her grandfather's death. The old man had died on a respirator, a victim of myasthenia gravis; the newborn baby had serious difficulty breathing and had to be placed on a respirator for the first week of his life. Was this merely coincidence, or a physical carryover?

Fortunately, Leslie's baby overcame his early problems and grew to be a healthy little boy. "He gives me great comfort and happiness," she says, "and whether imagined or not, I find the gap now closed that I had lived with all these years after my Grandpa died."

25

Listen to the Children

I thought everyone had these experiences until I mentioned them casually to my mama one day…

—*Joy**

Joy's story is all too typical. As a child, she saw colors around people and was aware of spirits, including a "pretend" playmate. When she talked about these things at the age of eight, her mother (perhaps frightened that her child might be abnormal) told her she was imagining them or making up a story. Joy learned to doubt herself and never to speak of her perceptions, until she discovered they were valuable assets in her work as a nurse and midwife.

I hear from many people who, as children, remembered pre-existence or sensed presences that the grownups couldn't see. Many of them tell of having been shut down by disbelief or even punishment. What a sad waste of children's natural gifts! If nothing else, I hope these stories will encourage parents to listen when their children say unusual things, and not discount everything as pure imagination.

From the time they begin to talk, children often express memories of birth, the womb, pre-existence, past lives, and even an awareness of their purpose in life. Why do we so easily shut them off? Novelist Danielle Steel's son Nick suffered from bipolar disorder and eventually committed suicide. When he was less than three years old, he told his mother a mysterious story. Her account of the incident illustrates some of the reasons people shy away from their children's startling revelations:

> He used to tell me interesting stories when he was small. He would go on for hours sometimes, just talking about things. And it was during one of these talks that he looked at me pensively one day, and began what he was saying to me with "When I was big…" and then he went on and told me a long story. I couldn't help asking him what he meant by what he had said. "What do you mean, 'when you were big'?" It seemed an odd thing for a child to say, and a little eerie, and it unnerved me, but he explained with a thoughtful look, as though trying to remember something.
>
> "I used to be big a long time ago, and now I'm small again. But when I was big…" He went on again then, while I watched him, and then he looked up at me oddly. "I used to be here before," he said quietly, "and I was big then." It was certainly an odd thing to say, and I didn't question him again. It made me too uncomfortable, and touched on things I didn't want to know.[1]

Children Have Memories of Other Lives

If we ignore their past life memories, we tend to have an idealized image of children as perfect, untainted beings. The reality of children is more interesting and less innocent. Can you imagine being a two-year-old who remembers dying as an adult at the hands of murderers—and who wants revenge? This is just one of the thoroughly documented cases in Dr. Ian Stevenson's *Children Who Remember Previous Lives*. As a toddler, this child was still angry about that death, until eventually the memory faded.

It's comforting to believe that death will dip us in purifying light and wash away all the negatives of a lifetime, and it's tempting to see newborn babies as embodiments of innocence. But research by Ian Stevenson and Carol Bowman, among others, reveals that this view may be too simplistic. Babies have emotional histories, and they bring baggage with them.

Some children retain past life memories for years, but more commonly they fade from conscious awareness around the age of six. Perhaps it is meant to be this way, so the distracting memories will not interfere with fully engaging in our new life. In one of Dr. Stevenson's cases, a little boy had such compelling memories of his previous life that he had trouble adjusting to the present reality. He kept longing to go and live with the previous family where he, or rather his former identity, had a wife and several grown-up sons. But even in this case, the memories finally faded away.

Knowledge of a Life Plan

Young children sometimes reveal an awareness of their own future. Psychologist Jan Hunt recalls her little boy commenting one day, "I'm supposed to live a very simple life." More sobering is the case of the English cellist, Jacqueline du Pre. As a child of about ten, she informed her sister, "When I grow up, I won't be able to walk or talk." Her phenomenal career was cut short in her twenties by the onset of multiple sclerosis, and ultimately she was indeed unable to walk or talk.[2] Could she have retained in childhood a fragment of a life plan made before birth?

Kathy: Something was familiar about this

When I was about three years old I was with my father and grandfather in Indiana. We had taken my grandpa's old red Ford pickup truck to the grocery store and we walked around a corner and there was a lady pushing twin babies in a stroller. I remember my father saying, "Oh look, isn't this special! Those are twins. She had two babies instead of one."

I remember standing there and looking at them for some time. Something was really familiar about this. I didn't say much the rest of our time in the store and remember standing in the middle of the pickup seat (long before child restraint laws) all the way back to the farm house and pondering the twins.

By the time we got there, I knew what it was. My grandpa and my dad were headed off to the barn when I went running after them yelling, "I'm going to have twins! Me too! I'm supposed to have twins!" They turned around and said, "Oh, that's nice" and just kind of laughed at me and brushed me off. I got real mad and stomped my feet on the gravel and pouted, "I am so supposed to have twins! You'll see!"

My girls are fourteen and identical twins. They look just like me and people frequently joke and call us triplets. I have no other children.

Knowledge of Babies On the Way

Children show their openness to the soul world in many ways, including a remarkable knowledge of babies yet to be born. In Chapter Nine, Miriam's little boy announced that a baby girl was living in their house, and asked whether Miriam could ever see her. Children somehow perceive the presence of souls whether before conception or during pregnancy—and not just their own brothers- and sisters-to-be. In the following story from South Africa, Tanja's invisible pregnancy is detected by a child who is a complete stranger to her:

Tanja: The boy at the airport

When I was seven weeks pregnant, we were at the airport to say farewell to friends of ours going overseas. A little boy whom I had never seen before said to his mother, "That lady over there is pregnant." I definitely did not show at that time! His mother, a bit embarrassed, told him to keep quiet. I then said to her that it is true and I am pregnant and how could he have possibly known this. She mentioned that from time to time he sees things. I asked him if he could see what sex the baby was and without hesitation he said it was a boy. Later in the pregnancy we went for a scan to determine the sex of the baby. I felt that if I knew, I could communicate with the baby better and also start using the name we had chosen for him/her. The scan showed that the baby was indeed a boy!

Kristy's small son kept track of an unborn sibling over time. Without ever being told of Kristy's pregnancies and miscarriages, he was aware of the soul in its comings and goings.

Kristy: "Baby will come back"

December 1998

I became pregnant with my first child four years ago, and while napping in the first weeks of pregnancy, I could feel her presence. She was warm and joyful, and seemed to embrace me. This pregnancy ended in miscarriage at seven weeks, and I felt the most profound grief of my life. I missed my "little girl," and still do.

Six months later, I became pregnant again. After reading the results of my home test, I walked around in the back yard on a lovely spring morning. I closed my eyes and meditated, to see if I could connect with this baby. Although I didn't feel the child's presence, a voice from inside seemed to say that this was a different child, a boy, and not my daughter of the previous pregnancy. I went on to give birth to my beautiful son, Alan.

Since Alan turned a year old, I've started feeling the presence of my first baby, the same loving, joyful presence I felt in that pregnancy. At home, I catch glimpses of a child in the corner of my eye. Sometimes, when we enter our home, after everyone is inside and I close the door, I feel like I left someone outside. I sometimes feel compelled to open the door and look.

I had a "conversation" with my miscarried daughter last summer. There seemed to be a voice from inside while I sat quietly. She seemed to tell me her time was running out, and that I needed to become pregnant soon. I told her I didn't think there was enough of me to go around for two children at the time; the idea overwhelmed me. I asked if the end of the year was too late to start, and this seemed all right to her.

Now that it is December, my husband and I feel ready to have another child. Alan has matured a lot from two-and-a-half to three years old, and his needs are more easily met by my husband and a few others. We made our first attempt at conceiving a child nine days ago. I feel like I am pregnant, not only with the early symptoms of pregnancy, but intuitively so. We are very hopeful! Last week at the dinner table, Alan said over and over, "My sister…my sister," not with any excitement or distress, just in his normal tone of voice. We don't make a habit of talking about babies or a sister. Once or twice in the last year I have asked him if he wants a brother or sister, but that is all.

January 1999: Yep, I'm pregnant! I'm about five weeks along. I feel like this is my girl, but no strong messages or voices have told me so, at least not yet. This past month, Alan has been saying, "My sister turned into a baby. In Mommy's tummy." Honest…with no prompting from anyone! He said this to my mother last week when we visited her. She was stunned!

Kristy was to lose this pregnancy in the first trimester. Little Alan seemed to know about it before being told—and even before the miscarriage was evident to Kristy.

This pregnancy was difficult for me. I had a feeling early on that all was not right. I couldn't connect with the baby—it was like I couldn't "find" him/her. I am doing fine physically, but need time to grieve and get the courage and mindset to be pregnant again. We are hoping to try again in the summer or fall.

My son's comments always amaze me. At six weeks, he told me the baby "went bye-bye." I started spotting a few days later. When I started my miscarriage, and told him that the baby was dead, he told me he was sorry, and then said, "Baby will come back." I like to think he has a special link to the child who may someday join our family.

April 2000

I am happy to say I am pregnant again, twenty-five weeks along and everything seems to be going well! Alan was right on the mark with this pregnancy, too. We weren't planning to tell him about it right away, but at four weeks gestation, he asked me if there was a baby in my tummy!

Baby Summer was born in July and Kristy reports, "I feel sure my daughter is the soul I conceived six years ago. She feels so much like she did during my first pregnancy, joyful and peaceful. It seems to me that she still knows of our history together, and knows she waited a long time to be here, just by how she looks at me sometimes, like she is still a wise old soul fresh from the divine."

Memories of the Womb and Before

Children often reveal memories of an existence before birth, both in the womb and in another realm. It is puzzling that a few people keep these memories in conscious awareness as they grow up, while most of us lose touch with them in childhood. Even parents who actively encourage sharing and holding onto prenatal memories are apt to see them fade by the age of six or seven. This fading seems to be a natural process, and I don't think we should strive to keep our children's memories active. Instead, I suggest making a written record of their revelations and saving it for them.

When children talk of "heaven," or "where I was before," they often describe playful, childlike scenes and activities—an odd contrast to the mature tone of so many pre-birth communications. Adults sharing soul memories invariably stress that it's nearly impossible to put that state of being into words; how much harder it must be for children, who haven't mastered a big vocabulary! To express something of their memories, they may have to use the simple, down-to-earth images available to them.

In their descriptions of where they were "before," children tend to name familiar religious and cultural figures. A mention of Jesus, angels, or God will catch our interest, making these the most likely memories to be noted and recorded. "Parent-friendly" memories of choosing mommy and daddy—these too are apt to be treasured. The content most compatible with our own ideas is easiest to accept, and tends to dominate the stories that are kept alive in family lore, while bizarre and unfamiliar comments may slip through the net of our attention and be lost.

I've even caught myself editing children's memory stories, wanting to drop details that don't fit my expectations. For example in the next story, young Jason mentions the "dead fish" in describing pre-exist-ence; I nearly deleted this puzzling note. In fact, it's the incongruous memories that may prove most revealing. As we listen to children, we need to make an extra effort to take in comments that are hard to grasp or make us uncomfortable.

Jennifer, a mother of two from Washington, kept a journal of the unusual things her son Jason told her about life before birth. Jason realizes that his memories have begun to slip away, and hopes his baby brother will refresh them as soon as he is able to talk well enough.

Jason was two and a half when Jennifer became pregnant again. He was very excited about the new baby, so Jennifer dreaded having to tell him when she miscarried early in the pregnancy:

Jason and "The Cupid Place"

> I explained that the "baby seed" inside of Mommy was sick and that it wasn't growing right and the baby would have to go back to God. And Jason told me, "Then it will just take longer to get born." He took in the information and walked out of the room, then he came back a minute later to say, "That baby wasn't here yet, it can just stay with God till it gets born. It's okay, God's a cool guy."

Soon after the miscarriage, Jennifer was pregnant again.

> I finally told Jason about the new baby (I had been waiting till we were sure this one would stay). He just smiled and said, "I know."
> Since he has known the baby is coming, Jason has been talking a lot more about where he was before he was born. Today he was

telling me about "The Cupid Place" (this is the first time he's given it a name) "where the babies have wings and play on clouds." He says he was there and that the babies "fall down from the sky into their Mommy's tummies" and he was helping "drop them down in." He explained that the King Cupid is God and he would come and "watch and talk to me" and he's a pretty nice guy. And that there was a big castle "kinda like our school" and that he could see me and Daddy and our house. He was telling me that most of the other babies were still little but he was two most of the time.

He complained he liked it better there than here and I told him I did too, even if I couldn't remember much, and that we'd get to go back again some day. He has told me about watching Daddy and me go to work and choosing us and the clouds and castles and seeing the planets and the "dead fish." I have no clue about the dead fish but he almost always brings it up when he talks about The Before.

He has told me about being in my womb too. "It was like being in space, I floated around a lot and it was red and I could hear you and Daddy and Socks (the dog) and I could hear the music and I danced in there and was upside down a lot." He said the water is salty in me and he could tell when I ate cookies because he could taste them. He gets this dreamy look when he talks about it. He has said babies cry when they're born because it hurts. I told him it's not supposed to hurt and he said, "They hurt my head when they pulled me out." (He knows he was pulled out with forceps because he has seen the video of his birth.)

I love these talks and I try my best not to prompt him and just let him ramble about it but sometimes I do have questions. I'm always afraid that because he misses being there so much he will try to go back early. I don't think I could deal with that.

It's a brother! Jason was so excited to finally meet his brother. He was right there with him after he was born, hugging and kissing him and trying to show him how to nurse. Any time anyone asks Jason if he was surprised it was a boy, he just smiles and tells them no, he knew it was a brother. He told me he played with him in the clouds before he was born.

I hope that parents are becoming more attuned to really listen to the amazing things our children tell us. We can learn so much!

Julie M. tells the story of her first grandchild, Gabrielle. She says, "I am convinced that Gabrielle is a very old soul. She shows a kindness and compassion that is rarely seen in a child."

Gabrielle: The little girl who missed her wings

As a baby, Gabrielle giggled at walls and babbled to the air. She laughed constantly. We were beginning to think the house was haunted! When Gabrielle was about thirty months old, she began pointing in the air and waving, especially in the car. When she started to talk, she insisted she was talking to her old friends, the angels. She questioned us as to whether we could see them.

Around age three, she began telling us things about Jesus. I had a crucifix in the living room and she told everyone, "That is *my* Jesus." Gabrielle says she was an angel and Jesus asked her to come here and be Tonya and Gabe's daughter because they will need her help. She tells stories of living in heaven and how her love for Jesus keeps happiness in her heart. Almost all of the incidents happened before Gabrielle ever was exposed to the church. We used to call her our little prophet because she preached to us about what Jesus expects from us before she was four years old.

Once, she ran through the living room, took a great leap and hit the floor. She had a surprised look on her face and started to laugh. "I forgot, I don't have wings anymore." Gabrielle often talked about her wings; she missed them very much, but Jesus promised her that after she came here to help Tonya and Gabe she could have her wings back when she returned.

Gabrielle got into a little trouble at Sunday school when she first started there. The teacher was telling the story of Noah's Ark. Gabrielle, four years old, promptly corrected the teacher about her version of the story. She told her she was telling the story wrong; she knew because she was there.

Gabrielle's baby sister Abigail was born when she was four. I called Abby a little angel once and Gabrielle corrected me. "Nani, I was an angel before I came here, but Abigail is just a little soul. People cannot be angels, and angels can only be people when Jesus asks them to. Like me."

Julie reports that by the age of seven and a half, Gabrielle has completely forgotten her earlier accounts of being an angel. "The really strange thing," says Julie, "is that she doesn't recall any of the stories she told, even the ones she told repeatedly."

Children Speak Startling Wisdom

Even before they are able to talk, children may find a way to reveal something of their far-reaching awareness. From Puerto Rico, Luz describes the surprising actions of her twelve-month-old baby, Gabriel. She was reading aloud a book about world religions. In the section on religions of India, she came across an unfamiliar word that sounded funny in Spanish. She and her husband laughed, whereupon Gabriel looked at them and said "No." Luz recalls:

> He stood up in front of us, opened his arms, looked to the sky, bowed, put his arms together in a praying position, looked down and then continued playing. At the same time he was doing this he was babbling something. After a while I asked him if he knew this religion and he said yes.
>
> He is only two now but there are times when I look at him and know I can ask him anything. Once I asked him if he knew me from before. He said yes and also yes to knowing my sister but he said he didn't know my husband. It's all a matter of knowing the correct time to ask, and by looking at him you can tell.

When children manifest a wisdom that they haven't learned in their present lifetime, perhaps they are releasing fragments of soul memory. In the following story, a child expresses transcendent knowledge—just before forgetting it all.

Lesta Bertoia: "We are all so conscious"[3]

When my son Eric was four, he made up a chant. "I love you, Ma, whole wide as the world," he would say, and then he would start singing. "I love you and you love me, just on the way…to heavenly light. We love each other, just on the way…to heavenly light." Heavenly light. From where he'd remembered that, I couldn't guess. When he was ten, he told me from where.

He was sitting on the floor among his Legos, gazing into some other dimension, when he started speaking in a deepened, monotone voice. "We were brought here from another part of the Universe. Humanity was planted on this planet. But also, some of us have traveled here spiritually. We actually live long lives as spirits. Each human lifetime is equal to one day in the life of who we are as spirits. Human lifetimes can go on for billions of years, but that is still only a small amount of time in the lifetime of a spirit. One spirit can expand to include many beings. It can even expand to include the whole Universe. It is hard to be in this body and to do the homework I have to do to fit in, but I have to do it so that I will appear to belong, and so that I can fulfill my purpose. I am starting not to be able to remember who I am. Time is Life and Life is Time and Death is Life and Life is Death."

The next day I asked him about what he'd said. He didn't know what I was talking about. He'd known it was about to happen, and it did. He'd forgotten. But he had helped me to take seriously what my daughter, who is seven years younger, had said when she was little.

Two years before Fawni was born, I had two abortions with her father within a few months. I was using birth control, but something more powerful than spermicide was at work, and yet, we just weren't ready. He needed to spend a year with another woman. I was already a single mom, and I needed to spend a year re-collecting myself.

We got back together, not even really sure why, until one day he put his arms around me and said, "Let's make a baby." My eyes grew wide. "For real?" I was so ready for this to happen. "Yeah." Neither time before had I experienced a knowing of conception, but this time, even before the normal signs showed up, we both knew who was on the way. As we sat in front of the woodstove one evening, we each saw, at the same time, with our third eye, a young woman in her twenties who looked a little like his sister and a little like my sister.

When she was two, our daughter asked me, "'Member, Ma, when I was up in de sky and I decided to be a little girl and come in your body?" I didn't even remember her ever having used the word *decided* before. When she was two and a half, I overheard her singing to herself in the bathtub. I was out in the hall, putting away the towels, and I paused in awe, hardly believing my ears. "We are all so conscious. We know everything. But we just like to play along. We are all so conscious. But we like to play."

I shouldn't have been surprised. By then she'd already been telling me about her past lives. "I was in a boat wif my baby and de on'y man I loved. We had a house in Canyafornia."

When she was three, she asked me about her cousin, "How come I'm the same age as her, Ma? I wanted to be older than her." "How much older, Fawni?" I asked. "Two years," was her response. She had obviously planned on arriving two years before we were ready. When she was in tenth grade, however, she remarked that she was glad she was the age she was, because she knew no one in the higher grades that she could relate to as well as she could to her closest friends, who were all in her grade. Now that she is nearing twenty, her father and I, who both feel blessed by her presence in our lives, see the same young woman we saw that night by the woodstove.

26

Haukie and Melissa

In each of the next three chapters, we'll explore soul communication in the context of a single family's life. These are families whose daily lives are entwined with colorful threads of soul connections. We'll follow them over time to see how their experiences play out, and what it is like to live with such openness to these mysteries.

The first story is about the lines of love from one generation to the next, and across the borders of life and death. It's the story of a little boy whose soul sense is unusually open and who seems aware of realities that are invisible to most of us. We follow the surprises of life with Hauk for more than a year and a half, while his mother, Melissa, travels a bumpy road toward bearing her second child.

March 2000

It wasn't until the birth of my son Hauk a year and a half ago that I really started to grieve for my mother, after twenty-seven years. She died when I was seven. I know that my dad dreams with her often. Knowing this, and finally angry with her one day, I started shouting at her. I screamed at her for leaving me alone to go through all the hell I have been through in my life, angry that she was not here to help me parent, angry that she showed herself to Dad and not to me. I really let her have it, sobbing and out loud. I felt foolish.

Next morning a book flew off the bookcase. It was on the top shelf behind a few others, and you had to wiggle it past the molding to get it on there. It was a book she used to read to me! I casually put it back in its place, and an hour later it came off again. For

221

a few days strange things like this were happening, and my husband was getting a little scared. So I told Mom, out loud, that the message was received but Rob was going to move if it happened again. It stopped.

About a month ago, I asked to meet her in my dreams, and I did! In the dream she reassured my of my parenting, and that she was near, and then she said I would have a beautiful baby girl. She said she would be the jewel of my husband's eye, his little gem. I awoke thrilled, not only to talk with Mom, but for the news, as we have been trying to have another baby.

Two weeks later, upon falling asleep, I saw a tiny, peaceful, happy little face float down and greet me as if to say hello. I know this is my next child; I felt it instantly. But I am suddenly impatient. I am finding myself apologizing to this child for scaring her away, left wondering if she is afraid to come for some reason. Am I being silly to question? Do others feel this way? My first child did not come easily and I feel the clock ticking, as I'm thirty-four.

April

Right as I was drifting off last night again, all of a sudden a little girl in pigtails, with a blue and white thin horizontal stripe shirt, stood standing there looking up at me, a little sad it seemed. My first thought was that it was me, but as I looked at her, I could see my husband in her, just like our son now. I turned my head in my sleep and she was gone. I tried to call to her and tell her I was all right (I was sick all day yesterday), and eventually I heard giggling, the giddy laughter of a child.

I think this is so great! And even greater that I can talk to someone about it! The excitement of meeting in dream state has made the anticipation of getting pregnant a little more bearable for me.

I'm afraid you will think I am a crackpot, but I also believe that Hauk is my grandfather come back. Time will tell as he grows; I wait with open eyes and ears to see what he has to say as he begins to talk. As he began getting into my kitchen drawers and things, he had a particular fondness for certain items. My grandfather was a baker and I have his old tools, pie crust crimpers, cookie cutters, cake decorators and so forth, mixed in the same drawer with my Mom's things as well as my newer stuff.

Hauk always grabs Grandpa Frank's things, takes off with them and sometimes hides them. He doesn't go much for Mom's or mine, just Grandpa's. It was kind of a joke and we kept calling him "baker Frank." He has shown a very special relationship with my father, which Dad and Grandpa had too.

July

Since Haukie's birth I've miscarried once, possibly twice (very early the second time). I was hospitalized twice for issues related to these, and needless to say, I am very frustrated with my situation. The fertility specialist says we need to try harder!

Hauk, now twenty-one months old, keeps saying he is going to have a sister. I have still been having dreams, but of two babies most recently. They seem to be about seven or eight month fetuses, strange to me. Perhaps they are the two I have lost. It could just be my way of sorting through what has been happening. I still sense the little girl very strongly, her features still vivid and close.

November

Hauk has been talking to a baby. He was really puzzled with me that I couldn't see it one day. He was chattering away, and then he said "Bye bye" to the baby. He kept asking me where the baby went. On several other occasions he has tried to point the baby out to me. How I wish I were open as children are!

But I can still so vividly see that little girl whom I have seen on the edge of sleep. I get the sense that she is just happily waiting to come here, and I should just be patient. I used to be the most patient person in the world—what happened?

Hauk woke up really scared one night and wanted to come sleep with us, that was a first. Then next afternoon, when he went in for a nap, he kept saying, "Mom, no ghost today, right? Go nite nite, no ghost?" I asked, "Did you see someone last night?" He said, "Yes, papa ghost." I'm interpreting that to mean an older gentleman, as all older people are papas (grandpas).

February 2001

I had another miscarriage in December, but some interesting things surrounded it. Hauk was telling me that there was a baby around shortly before I found out I was pregnant. Eventually one day he pointed to my tummy and said, "Baby." We don't know any other pregnant women that he would have associated it with. Then I found out I was pregnant, about two and a half months along.

One day Hauk started telling me that he was sorry, baby went bye bye. When I asked him where baby went, he said, "Up" and floated his hands up as if to show me how. I remember thinking, "Oh god, no…don't tell me he knows something before I do." Sure enough, two days later I miscarried. I really didn't speak to Hauk about any of it, not about being pregnant or the miscarriage, just went about my day as usual. About a week and a half after I lost it, Hauk out of the blue said, "I'm sorry baby died, Mom, I'm sorry," and he kissed me, my "boo boo." I was astounded. There is no doubt in my mind that Hauk was fully aware of all of it, even though not a word was spoken on the subject.

Hauk has also been talking quite often to "ghosts," as he calls them (a word I don't use). He was even calling out to one yesterday as he looked through the house. On occasion he gives me a message from them: "Ghost says hi, Mom." "Oh, okay, honey, tell them I said hi too." He said he saw angels flying in my bedroom one day as we took our nap together; he chuckled and giggled as he pointed to one, following it about.

We'll be driving down the road and he'll start talking about a dog he sees, he'll say the color and so on, and I don't see it. Until about a mile down the road we finally come upon it, and he says, "See, Mom, there he is." He will describe a house we are going to when it is miles away yet and unseen. I really enjoy the things Haukie comes up with, and I try so hard not to feed into it, or deny it. I just take it all as naturally as possible. My poor husband gets a little scared, though.

June

Hey! I have good news for a change, I'm pregnant! I'm only about three and a half months along now, but baby has made it through an emergency appendectomy that I had a few weeks ago. If "she" made it through surgery, I suspect this one may be a keeper! And I'm sick as heck, and not complaining. Hauk is firm in his belief that it is a girl; we'll know in a sonogram in a couple of weeks.

We've had almost weekly sonograms with this one for various reasons.

My little angel Hauk has again been coming up with some interesting things. He has been talking a great deal about "Grandma" who visits here almost daily. He'll begin talking to her in his room when we are there, but as soon as I start asking vague questions, he gets all shy. We've been asking him what we should name the baby, but he hasn't said yet.

Before I knew I was pregnant, I overheard him singing in his bed at naptime one day. In his own little melody, he was singing of a naked baby coming down and being in the tummy, and he also was saying that Grandpa was there while baby came down. It was really sweet, and I didn't think much of it at the time, for I had pretty much given up on getting pregnant at that point.

Then one night at dinner, after my first sonogram, he was telling his dad about it and how he saw the baby. Mind you, we watch almost no TV, nor do we talk to him of pregnancy and birth. He swiftly started telling my husband that "Baby get big, and doctor will pick Mom's shirt up, cut off her boobs and pull the baby out." Okay, so they didn't actually cut "them" off during my C-section, but it sure sounded to us like Hauk was recalling his entrance into this world almost three years ago. We had to chuckle, a little astonished at what he was explaining.

I still swear Hauk can astral project around at night, and see things ahead. He has this knowing of so many things that I know we didn't talk about in front of him. I had a dream the other night where in mid-dream I said, "Hey, are you in my dream, or am I in yours, we're both in the same dream, isn't this cool!" He giggled and agreed. It was very lucid and the neatest thing I have experienced. Hauk is extremely empathetic and open; I hope it continues for a long time. He took such good care of me while I recovered from surgery it was amazing.

August

Mom and Hauk were right, it's a girl! We tried to tell Hauk that the doctor said it was a boy; he said, "No, it's my sister, not a boy, a girl baby!" Hauk then said I must have another baby after the girl, *that* will be his brother.

Baby Isabella was safely born in December. Hauk, who has been talking more and more about past life memories, continues to maintain that his brother will eventually join the family too. Melissa isn't so sure she's up to it!

27

Anne's Story

I sometimes grin at myself, trying to glimpse the answers to the questions of the ages by looking through just the one small window I have, that of soul-to-soul family relationships.

—*Anne*

For over three years, Anne* has shared her unique experiences and insights with me. I've learned much, especially about the art of listening to our children. Her story is a still-unfolding adventure with a trio of souls she first met as a child. We shall begin by getting to know her and her husband Paul,* as well as Anne's mother, who plays an important part in the story. At the beginning of our acquaintance, Anne and Paul have one child, Gabriel, just two years old. Anne writes:

> My mother had a rough childhood and also a rough adulthood in some ways, but however difficult things were for her, she gave me some great gifts. She had us learn to meditate, taught us to do self-hypnosis, analyze our dreams, and to think and argue philosophically. She was into psychology, and brought home interesting things to do. I learned a lot about myself and how to analyze my own feelings.
>
> The self-analysis came in handy, since I was raped when I was seven. I didn't deal with it until I was fourteen, didn't even tell my mom until I was in my twenties. I had a year of therapy, and while

I still get some bad stuff coming off echoes of it, I'm basically sane and healthy, but wiser for the whole set of experiences.

I draw on both my Native American and Celtic roots for my spiritual imagery. I have had moments of astounding awareness and insight, and moments of clear vision, and moments that terrified me...And I spend the rest of my life just like everyone else, stumbling around and through, struggling with daily stuff and trying to remain positive and energetic. I have a master's degree in Human Geography; my current job is as a technical writer. I love being helpful to others, and I love debate as long as it stays respectful.

Paul was the first guy I ever met who did not have to learn to respect women. He grew up respecting women. He is a systems-engineer-type, with the "I believe what I can prove, or what I can reasonably extrapolate" approach. But he respects my opinion and my approach to life absolutely. His architecture designs often reflect a very deep spiritual understanding—one that he can seldom articulate, but which shows in the designs.

The Dream Playmates

I knew and played with my three sons (two yet to be born) when I was still a child. Around age seven, I had many recurring dreams of riding bikes with three boys who were my sons, even though they were about my age or older. The oldest boy was the most clear to me, and the other two didn't connect quite as strongly, though they were all firmly present.

I think they felt bad for me because I didn't have many friends, and I had recently been sexually assaulted by a distant family member. The innocent fun we had riding our bikes, and the slightly protective feeling I got from the oldest boy, helped me get through that time. I always thought the eldest was cute. He was also smart and thoughtful and took his responsibilities seriously, looking after his brothers and guiding our play. But he was still fun. The younger two were more free-spirited.

I always knew those playmates were my sons. It was an odd feeling, since I knew both during the dreaming and when I was awake that they were my sons and hadn't been born yet, and yet they were older than me. I just accepted the paradox the way kids accept things, but I knew that anyone else would find it strange.

I felt the kind of affection for them that one does for family. And there was an echo of maternal pride as well, because my sons were decent, loving, thoughtful, and fun kids, the kind I was happy to play with myself—and since they were boys, that was saying something! I remember being upset over the fact that they were boys and there were three of them, because I only wanted two children and I wanted daughters. I had my plans, but their presence overrode them. I simply came to accept that while I might want two kids, I was having three, and while I might want daughters, I was having sons.

When I met Paul, he thought three was a better number of kids, so there was that third child, not an accident after all. Knowing that all three boys were planned and wanted was very comforting, like a circle had closed, the other shoe had dropped, and the universe was congruous again.

Pregnant with Gabriel: Visions and Messages

When I was about three months pregnant with Gabriel, I saw him (the eldest) again. I had just woken up, and was enjoying a few moments of blissful sleepy time in bed while Paul was in the shower. I glanced down to the end of the bed, and there he was. Instead of being ten or eleven as usual, he was about three years old. He had straight smooth hair, light brown with reddish highlights (both Paul and I have dark hair). I couldn't see his eyes, because they were watching the little red truck he was zooming over the folds in the blankets. He was waiting, I could tell, and he was playing with his truck while he waited.

Paul came in the door just then, and the boy vanished. I swear I was awake, but when I tell people the story, I say it was a dream, unless they're the kind who would understand. The firmness of his age made me feel like he had last been a child at that age, as though he had died as a three-year-old. That made me a little sad, but I didn't think on it too much, since I was so excited to have seen him so clearly.

This sweet boy also has a close link to my best friend. The day I found out I was pregnant, she called me at work. She asked me if I had anything to tell her (I was waiting to tell people until the third month, and this was too soon). She said she had a dream so vivid that she felt like my baby boy (*boy!*) had called her on the phone to announce his presence, his sex, his appearance (blue eyes, wavy reddish hair), and his name. We didn't use the name he offered, but he doesn't seem to mind.

Near the end of the pregnancy, he also told my friend that I needed to eat more protein. She called me up and told me I needed more protein for the baby. I ate more, but not enough more. Three weeks later, my blood pressure started to rise, and my midwife told me I wasn't getting enough protein—the baby needed more! I had to smile sheepishly, because I'd been told even before the problem was noticeable, but I hadn't taken it seriously enough. When I ate enough protein (lots) my blood pressure dropped back to normal.

Gabe had a pre-birth visit with one of my sisters, too. He sure got around! And he has a strong angel keeping an eye on him. I've seen strange things like a heavy swinging door *pause* in the process of swinging closed on him, giving him just enough time to get through instead of being crushed. I am not an "angel" person, but I had an angel helping me through eighty hours of back labor, and my mother swears the dim birth room lit up when he was born.

By the way, Gabriel has blue eyes and light brown hair with strong red highlights, to the point that some pictures of him make him look like a total carrot-top! And his straight hair turns wavy when it gets wet, but straightens when it dries. So all the images of him were spot-on.

I didn't really remember past lives as a child, I just knew they were there. Several times I told my mom that "when I was *your* mommy, I never made you do…(whatever)." I knew I was fudging, at least about making her clean her room, but I also knew I had been her mommy. And I knew I would be her mommy again. Another quote was, "When I'm your mommy, I'll let you do…" I used this as bribe material, trading favors, but I knew it was true. I was quite aware of the choice process, too. When talking to Mom about why she had seven kids, I remembered the lines of people waiting for each mother. She and I both knew that her children chose her.

My mother felt strongly that her first child was a teacher, who came to her on purpose. Her parents were abusive and didn't understand children at all, so she had no good role models. Her first child, when she was a newly married eighteen-year-old, had hydrocephaly. Grant was born "normal" and developed a fluid buildup in his brain soon afterwards that crushed his development. His IQ was very low as a result, and he had other problems.

But his ability to love was paramount. Grant loved his mommy absolutely. And he reacted to her parenting like a normal child, except that he didn't retain any of it. She could see her mistakes take hold in him, but by the next morning the slate was clean again. She learned what was right and wrong by watching his reactions to what she did. He molded her parenting to a quite decent model. And as soon as she was a good mother, he died of spinal meningitis contracted through the external shunt. He was three years old. She has a picture of him sitting in the corner of the sofa, laughing. It is up on the wall with the rest of our pictures, and I just noticed last week that Gabriel looks a lot like Grant, though I don't think they are the same soul.

As for the boys I met as a child, I've tried to see the younger two recently—I'd like to get to know them better before they come. I did it through a meditation: I was hoping to see them, and asked them to be there. I have done guided meditation for years, and can go into a trance state very easily. My visions are not "controllable," that is, I can follow a general path, but the details come as they please and not as I would choose them.

Meditating for images does not produce the crystalline clarity of a visitation for me; it is more like talking to someone through a closed window. On the other hand, when a vision comes unbidden, it is sharp, loud, and *close*. I feel like I could touch it. It feels real. A meditation vision is more like a daydream that has its own plan.

And according to this meditation vision, the boy who was to be second is having second thoughts. He isn't sure that he wants to be second to Gabriel. I got the sense he's worried I won't love him as much, and he'll always have to measure himself against his brother. The youngest is a pleaser-type, who tries hard to make up for the lacks in others. I promised to do my best to treat everyone fairly, and assured them I would have enough love to go around equally. That mollified the middle one a bit, but he still wasn't solid.

Journal of a Short Pregnancy

December 1999

OOPS. Started taking prenatal vitamins just in case. We weren't planning this timing, but it will work. We can't see taking action to abort or doing the "day after" pills since we know we are able and reasonably ready.

12/18

Company Holiday party. Feel really happy, in love with life, joyful, and at peace. When I tell Paul this, he says: "You are definitely pregnant!" I laugh. Implantation should be in the next two to four days if it happens.

12/21

Had a wonderful dream vision of meeting the soul of this child. About two A.M., I woke to a sense of something else present. Very hard to describe, because it was nothing I have ever seen or felt before. A light "being," in front of me, about the size that your arms make when you hug someone. In form, round but not round, spherical but not spherical. A perfect shape, but not one I can easily describe. The closest is if you stuck your head inside a giant balloon, so that the larger part was in front of your eyes: you know it is a sphere, but you can't see the whole thing.

The color was neither bright nor dark, but blazing in some sense that was not seen with my eyes. Almost like an eclipse, but the dark center was soft gray, and the edge was a gentle enough light to look at easily. The concept of halo works best, like a moon-dog or spectrum shift around a star.

I was flooded with a sense of peace, joy, bliss, and love. I knew immediately that this child would be one of incredible joyfulness, one I could easily love as much as I love Gabriel.

12/31

Miscarried this morning. Now I know why I stopped feeling pregnant, even when the symptoms continued. No goodbye from that soul, but a sense that it was gone. I am a little disappointed about the loss, but not sad exactly. It would be more painful if we had been trying, or if it had been further along. It is more like the feeling I have over my best friend moving to England for a few years: I miss her, but I know I'll see her again. I miss that beautiful presence, but I don't feel the grief of a death. More of a parting.

Spring, 2000

I've felt the presence of that soul I met (and "lost") off and on for a few months now, still always over the left shoulder. Yesterday morning, it got into my head.

I was giving Paul the usual hug and smooch goodbye, and the thought "*How about a quickie?*" popped into my head. In writing! Now, I don't think in words like that, so it was really kind of funny. The experience was so peculiar, I had to laugh, and then I had to explain why I was laughing. It felt like the words were written there in my mind, and someone popped them up like a jack in the box. Now, I'm not much of a "quickie" person, and less so when I am short on hours for the workweek! So we chuckled, winked, and went our separate ways to work.

About mid-day, I noticed signs that I was at peak fertility. Just as I noticed this, I "heard" a merry, mischievous laugh from over my left shoulder. My instant reaction was Ah-HA! That thought this morning was from you, scamp! Trying to hurry us along, I bet. I told that merry little soul that it will just have to wait for everyone to be ready. It doesn't seem chastened at all, though. I think we're in for an interesting time with this one.

Does Gabriel Remember?

Gabriel is two and a half now. He may have given me a glimpse of recall from when he visited me in my childhood. We were driving home from my sister-in-law's house, and went through a patch of woods. He started talking about the trees, and I told him that a lot of trees together are called a forest. The rest of the conversation went like this:

Me: So, a lot of trees all together are a forest. I used to play in a forest when I was little—a very small forest we called Apache Forest.
G: (interjecting excitedly) Me, too! I played in Apa-chee forest *wiff* you.
Me: (trying not to have my antenna poke up too high) Really? When did you do that?
G: I was a…you a girl, uh, I…you little, uh…I big (sounding progressively more frightened, voice going up in pitch and volume) I play in Apa-chee…in-a forest with you! (fairly desperate sounding, and confused, nearly panic-level)
Me: (trying to be casual to let him calm down) That's nice, did we have fun?
G: Uh-huh. Look for cows? (definite relief at his change of subject.)

Not great material for identification purposes—he is very imaginative, and makes up stories about us all the time, and I did refer to myself as little, but:

1) he usually uses present or future tense for pretend stuff ("We go fly up in de sky in a space-ship mommy? Dat sound like fun?"), and uses past tense for "real" memories, like when he tells me about taking a walk with Daddy.

2) he is very certain of what is make-believe and what is not (I get scolded if I don't notice the difference: "I just '*tending*, mommy, it's just pe-tend!"), and he has a different voice for pretend and "real" memory. He uses a sing-song for pretend stuff, and this wasn't that voice, and

3) the major stress in his voice was not usual at all.

I've never mentioned the playing in the forest before; I actually hadn't remembered that "Apache Forest" was often the destination for our dreamtime bike rides. My memories focus more on the pauses in the ride, where I would rest and look at them, trying to keep them in my memory.
In my mind there is a fine line between listening well and hearing stuff that isn't there. I don't want to think I messed with the system (hearing something that wasn't there), but I know that even the act of observation changes the dynamics, so there you are, you

messed with the system! So I remember every detail I can, and check to see if I missed a simpler explanation, one that fits the "normal world" more closely.

I live every day in communication with another soul, or two, or three, or more. I know that my son Gabriel spoke to my friend, visited my sister, and provided a lot of support to me when I was little, all before he was born. And I know I can feel and sometimes hear my next son, hanging out over my left shoulder, sometimes that merry child-soul, sometimes the more subtle adult version, sometimes not present enough to notice, sometimes so "there" that I can feel the weight of his hand resting on my shoulder. My daily life is colored and shaded and reshaped by these experiences.

Believing these things is a paradox. Like faith, there is no proof other than the evidence of your personal experience. You can hear the tales of others, and shiver with delight and the terrifying awesome differentness of it all, and yet be completely comfortable and at ease with the same kind of thing happening to yourself, because *that* experience is familiar.

I cannot explain how it happened that my sons visited me long ago, or how I knew they were my sons-to-be, or why it doesn't happen to everyone else. Most of the time, explanation is the last thing I care about. Unless I am trying to tell my story to someone who hasn't experienced something similar, or who has rejected the tales of others, closing themselves to the possibility. I find I sometimes have to join them in saying "how strange, how weird," because from the perspective of the surface culture, these are strange and weird experiences. I've had people grin and relate similar experiences, or shudder and say "how scary" (frightening to think their world might be larger than they want to believe?), or pause, look down a moment, then look at me and say, "Now I have to rethink everything I believed about souls and afterlives and how children come into being." And sometimes I meet someone whose face lights up and who listens with eyes glistening, as full of awe and delight as I am.

Gabriel is almost three. My mother is certain now that he is the same soul as her first son, Grant. Here's why: First, Gabe has a different personality than all the other kids of the last two generations, except for Grant. Grant was intensely sweet natured, compliant, emotionally open and aware, and affectionate. So is Gabriel. Grant died when he was three. The time I "saw" Gabe while I was pregnant, he was three, and I felt somehow like that was the age he "stopped" at in his last life. Only one of the three boys in my dream visits felt really close and real, that being the eldest. He was very protective, and when Mom suggested maybe this was the same soul, it clicked—he felt like a big brother to me!

I was visited by the next boy again, this time as a young adult. In a dream, he introduced himself as Colin, specifically to help me pick a name for him, since I've been complaining that finding the right name for this next boy would be difficult. And what do you know? Colin works. I have had increasing contact with this one. He's a very companionable and loving guy, much more mature spiritually than I anticipated, given my limited contact with him in the childhood dreams.

Paul has proposed we start trying for child number two sooner than planned, and he suggested that maybe the soul has been working on him, too.

"The Round Thing with the Eggs is Gone"

I miscarried at the end of August, at almost eight weeks. I never had a real soul connection on this one, though I did have a very intense dream about giving birth to a girl on the sidewalk on the way to the birth center. She was beautiful, looked part African-American, had a delicious laugh, and was very there and centered. She laughed all the way from her soul when I picked her up from the sidewalk, and asked if I wouldn't rather "have" her inside? She had a beautiful smile, like the sun coming out. Together we re-ran the dream to allow me to give birth to her inside, though we still didn't make it to the birth center; instead I had her in a guest room of a friend's house. That was the only dream about pregnancy I had the whole time.

I had lots of signs that something wasn't usual, though I didn't know how to interpret them. I kept getting and then losing symptoms, then getting them back. I didn't feel pregnant, even though I had a positive test result. I wondered if I was blocking something, or what. Then I started to spot, and two days later, I miscarried completely.

On the day I started spotting, when I picked up my almost-three-year-old Gabe from daycare, he asked me how I was, which is unusual. I said I was a little sad, then tried to figure out what more to say, since I hadn't told him I was pregnant, and we had been careful not to say anything around him. He immediately piped up with: "Mommy, are you sad because the round thing with the eggs in it is gone?"

Whoa. I tried to get more information from him without leading questions. I asked him what round thing with the eggs in it. He replied, "*You* know, the round thing, with the eggs in it..." When I questioned him further, he got that scared look again, and switched to, "Cookies are round, too, and dey hab eggs in dem, maybe a cookie is missing?" Then he clammed up completely.

He wouldn't make eye contact after that for a bit. He acted kind of guilty, like he'd once again said something he wasn't supposed to. Still, I'm glad he said it. It helps to know that he knew already, since half my sadness was for him because he so wants a younger sibling. And he didn't describe a soul being gone, he described an embryo in an early sac, just exactly the stage (five weeks) where this embryo stopped developing according to the sonogram.

Not long after the miscarriage, I started talking to Gabriel about siblings. He kept saying he wanted a sister. A baby girl, a sister, a girl, a sister. When I told him that he didn't get to choose if it was a boy or a girl, he stared me straight in the eye and said, "I got to choose *last* time." And then he turned and walked away.

So we tried again. And I started getting pregnancy symptoms, stronger this time, more stable. The day they peaked, I saw a few friends, one of whom is a psychic. She said right away when she saw me, "You are pregnant, and it is a girl"– and I hadn't been planning on saying anything to her about it. The next day, my symptoms started declining. Either I misread the symptoms and had never been pregnant, or I had a failed implantation cycle, which is about 50% of all conceptions.

In the car that day, I mentioned to Gabriel that it might take a long time to make a little brother or sister for him. I asked him if he still wanted a sister more than a brother. He said emphatically, "Yes, I want a sister. A little girl baby." Then he paused, and blurted out: "Any baby is fine, if I just get a baby." Then he clammed up again, and looked out the window, refusing to make eye contact.

It sucked to have geared myself up again, and I didn't like feeling like I was making it all up. Someone suggested I call the friend who had said it was a girl, and see if she picked up anything else. So I did. She said: "Yes, you were pregnant, but she isn't supposed to be your child. Gabriel is lonely for her; they spent time together before he was born, and have been connected before that. She is drawn to you when he calls her, but she doesn't want to be his sister, so she leaves again."

Then she said, "You are not supposed to get pregnant until January or later. If you try, she'll get called again, and that isn't what is supposed to happen. Gabriel is three, and he can't stand the idea of waiting possibly years and years to be with her again. He misses her terribly and he wants her *now*. If you wait until January, she'll be unavailable, so then you can have the child you are supposed to have. You are supposed to have boys."

That evening, I got a call from another friend. She told me straight off without her usual preamble, that she strongly felt I needed to wait until next year, because something bad would happen if I tried before next year. She had this overwhelming sense that it was important, the feeling had just flashed into her mind and she needed to tell me. She was trying hard to convince me to say, yes, I'll stop trying until next year. That annoyed me, and it was only after I hung up the phone that I realized she had backed up what the first friend said.

Then I checked my e-mail, and another friend had sent me a note saying she thought I should hold off for two or three months and then just let things happen. She had a feeling that things would work out right if I stopped trying for a while. Okay, OKAY! I got the message! I told my husband about the overlapping messages, and he laughed with relief. He said he was glad someone else mentioned it, because he was afraid if he asked me to stop trying for a few months, I'd take his head off.

The next day, I called my mom, and she jumped right in before I got more than a few words out, saying that she felt I should stop trying for a bit. And then I got another e-mail from yet another friend, who said that maybe I should wait until after the holidays. How's that for getting beaten over the head with the same message?

So yes, we are not trying until January.

The hard part with listening to the stuff our kids say is filtering. Set the filter wrong and you either screen out too much or not enough. Gabriel also talks about being the daddy or the mommy, but part of that is just normal role-playing. It is when he is insistent or…well, there's something about how he says something that cues me. I don't know what it is, but I get the feeling that someone said "LISTEN!" Sometimes it seems like the whole world got quiet right before he says it, and sometimes I just get a sudden focus.

I think it also helps that he speaks so well for someone his age. With kids who speak later, there's less of a window when their inner knowledge and their outer language skills match up. It's a window of opportunity before the "real" world takes precedence over the world that society doesn't reinforce. I know that many parents kill off this content by saying their kids are lying, making up tales, or being silly. But I can tell when he's being silly and when he's being serious—and sometimes both at once.

Here's a recent conversation. It began at K-Mart when Gabriel spotted a cool-looking rocking motorcycle.

G: Ohh, look!
M: That's a baby toy, Gabriel. Look at the picture.
G: I'll get it for my baby brother.
M: You don't *have* a baby brother.
G: Can you make one for me? Pleeeese?
M: (grinning) We can try. But it takes a *long* time.
G: That's okay. I'll give this to him when he's here.
M: That's really nice. We'll have to remember to come back and get this for him when he's here.

We picked up the conversation again later, in his room.

Me: So, you want me to make a baby brother for you.
G: Uh-huh. Two.
Me: Two baby brothers?
G: No, one baby brother and one baby sister.
Me: Well, we'll see—we don't get to pick.
G: Okay. (First time he said okay to that concept!)
Me: So when do you think your baby brother will be here? It takes a long time. What do you think? Around your birthday? By Christmas? Around New Year? In the spring? In the summer?
G: Not around my birfday. Before Christmas. That's right.

I think you can see how hard it would be to filter this all the time. Was the "baby brother" because the toy he spotted was a "boy thing"? Or was it because he's really in the know? I don't know. But he was definite about the Before Christmas timing, and he also was definite when he told me that a friend of mine is having a boy. Funny, my friend believes him…

Paul has always taken my description of the dreams of my sons at face value. Between my not trying to force him onto my planet, and his being comfortable with the fact that my planet and his are different but truly equal, none of the soul connection stuff ever seems to bother him. He smiles and shrugs when Gabriel volunteers information that is beyond the norm—not that it's something to ignore, just normal for him.

For example, about a week ago, I heard Gabe on the back steps. He was singing out, "Here, catbird, *here*, catbird! C'mere, c'mere, catbird!" I stepped outside to see what he was up to. He was sitting on the step, watching a bird on the fence—a catbird, by the way. He kept calling to it, and it hopped closer, flying for short bits, cocking its head at him and singing back. It took me a moment to realize that it wasn't singing the usual catbird songs, but was making alternating "nesting chirps" and inquisitive sounds. It was answering! It hopped closer and closer, responding to him as he kept calling.

Unfortunately, I made some motion, and the catbird glanced at me in alarm and flew away. I felt bad about that; I wanted to know what the end point would have been, and I'd interrupted what was clearly a private conversation! I apologized to Gabe, and told him

I'd go back inside and he could call it again. He shook his head and said, "No, I can't call it again. It will get mad at me if I call it again, and then it won't be my friend anymore." He wasn't upset, he just knew what the rules were.

I looked through the door at Paul, who had seen parts of this, and indicated how stunned I was by the interaction between child and wild thing. Paul's response was, "Why are you surprised? He does this *all the time*—" in reference to the seals (who leapt from the water each time he called them), or the dolphins (who stopped leaping to poke their heads out of the water to look at him), or the fact that butterflies and dragonflies fly up and land on him, or that wild ducks bring their ducklings right up to him, or that once a feral cat came running to comfort him when he hurt himself and cried...

Spring, 2001

I guess I should have asked Gabriel if his "little brother" would be here before Halloween. I'm pregnant, and due on October 27th! Now, why didn't I ask about that date? Another thing that is tough with listening is asking the right questions.

I'm almost twelve weeks, and so far so good. Gabriel is flip-flopping about whether this is a boy or a girl, but he seems to be leaning toward "I want a girl, but it is a boy" statements. We'll see. No major dreams or other contacts, though the dreams I've had are definitely of boys. Gabe is being very cute about the whole thing, wanting to feed the baby when it is born, and putting his hand on my tummy and announcing that he felt it kick! You can't possibly feel it from the outside, yet!

In late October, Anne and Paul's second boy was born, healthy and beautiful. And so the adventure continues...

28

Emily and her Daughters

o o o o o o o o o o o o o o o o o o o o o o o o o o o o o o o o o o

We have a big back yard loaded with old trees and a brook running through the property. There are rocks covered with lush green moss scattered in the brook, and clusters of violets on the bank that catch the evening light and glow deep purple. Wisteria blossoms hang down and drag their toes in the water...

—Emily

When Emily* connected with me in the early spring of 2000, I met an unusual family. Emily is a writer, as you can tell from the passage heading this chapter; her husband Ted* is a photojournalist. Their daughters, Sophie and Rose, both show signs of the expanded awareness typical of children but easily overlooked by some parents.

Imagine for a moment that you were born into a family of people who never have dreams and don't believe that such things exist. But you are a strange little kid: you experience nightly visions in full color, seeing unknown people in unfamiliar landscapes and having adventures that sometimes delight and sometimes frighten you. Without validation from your family (they've told you to quit your crazy talk), what can you make of this other reality you often visit?

It must be somewhat like this for children who are open to non-physical dimensions but whose parents cannot relate to their experiences. Sophie and Rose are lucky; their parents provide them with a supportive, nurturing environment where their abilities can flourish. This chapter is a story of living with soul awareness over two years' time, and it illuminates both the difficulties and the gifts that arise from children's openness. At the beginning of the year, Sophie is five and baby sister Rose is just two. Emily begins:

> Our daughter Sophie started talking at a very early age, so we were privy to the way a young child thinks in a special way. Her first clear words, "thank you," came at three months. She started trying to spell at eighteen months.
>
> Sophie is psychic in many ways and seems able to read minds. She is always asking me to explain words that she doesn't understand, words that have just been in my thoughts. For instance the other morning I was driving her to preschool and thinking about my own mother and how unappreciated she must have felt at times. Sophie piped up with, "Mom, what's unappreciated?" I started trying to explain "appreciated" first, and she corrected me. "No, I mean *un*-appreciated." She also seems to know things from another time, things there is no way she could know now, for instance thinking she saw her old skate key when she was two years old.
>
> She has often talked about her "mommy's tummy" experiences, and refers to "two ghosts" who kept her company in there. She has brought them up ever since she could speak. One was named "Casper," and the other "Sally." This intrigues me because Sally was my grandmother's nickname. She says there were also angels, but they didn't talk with her, only the two nice ghosts, who told her about herself and what she would be like when she was born.
>
> As for the name Casper, I think it came after seeing the movie about the friendly ghost, but she has always talked about two "beings" who played with her in the womb. One was male, the other female. It was after seeing the movie that she grabbed onto the ghost idea, almost as if it was a relief to have a name for what she experienced.
>
> Sophie has communicated repeatedly with her paternal grandfather, who died when she was three months old. My husband, Ted, is intrigued and supportive. He was with Sophie and me when she had her first conversation with her grandfather. It happened when

she had just turned two. We were visiting my husband's mother and staying in what had been the grandfather's room. Sophie started to talk about her cousin Heather (Ted's niece he's been very close to), who was driving in to visit that night. She said that Grandpa was sitting right there and he didn't like "the man in the white tee-shirt." Heather arrived about an hour later, with a man wearing a white tee-shirt. Heather later broke up with the guy, and we learned he was emotionally abusive to her.

Is this sort of thing fairly common? I try to honor Sophie with it and not make a big deal out of it but also not belittle it or question it, in hope that she'll keep it up as a natural part of her being.

Oh help. It's Saturday morning and Sophie is pelting me with questions about everything on earth that she can think of. What does "I beg you" mean, for instance, and why can't we wake up her baby sister with ringing a dinner bell and what do I mean she doesn't know karate well enough to defend herself so she can stay alone at home while I go to the hardware store?

I just had an eerie realization. A few nights ago Sophie and her sister and I were having dinner and she announced that her Grandpa had something to say to us. She said something that was very Pop-like (about money; the man was obsessed with it). And then she said something about how she needed to keep saying "thank you."

When Sophie said "thank you" the first time, we were in Hawaii. My husband had an afternoon off and we were at an outdoor restaurant in Kona. A woman came over to our table to admire Sophie and asked how old she was. We told her three months and she started to coo at her some more. The woman was a real champion baby-cooer.

Sophie, clear as a bell, and I swear with an "enough, already!" tone to her voice, said, "Thank you." Whereupon the woman totally freaked out and said something about that being the smartest baby she'd ever seen and practically shrieked the whole way back to her table.

I knew absolutely nothing about babies. Never was around them. Had just turned thirty-eight, so I'd logged a lot of years never being around them. Speaking at three months didn't faze me, but it thrilled my baby-savvy spouse who immediately got up and called his dad from a pay phone to tell him. What just hit me is I think that was almost the last phone call with his dad, certainly the last important one that would sing out. Suddenly, her mentioning Pop talking about her saying "thank you" feels more significant.

I do believe in reincarnation and have had three channelers "read" Sophie. She has always been an unusual child and I felt that there was an intensity to her night-time fears that transcended what most children experience. All three channelers said she had been a young girl, aged fourteen or so, at Auschwitz. We aren't Jewish, but it somehow fits.

Everyone also said that Sophie was French, which was a feeling I have always had with her because she is so drawn to anything French. However, I speak the language and have worked in France, so Sophie might have just clued in to me.

To deepen her "French Connection" though, this past fall we were in the car and she piped up from the back seat about how she missed my jewel box from when I was her mommy before. This made my ears perk up. She said, "from when we lived before in France" and I had "that big jewel box" and she would go "like this," and I watched her in my rear view mirror make a grand scooping gesture, like a little girl might with a big box of necklaces. I am not much of a jewelry wearer in this life, so Sophie wasn't confusing our present experience with her thoughts. She spoke about that time for a few weeks after that, but then stopped.

My gut has always been tied to England, so much so that on various visits I have actually seen places I'd dreamed about, although my dreams were always in an earlier time. All of my "feelings" of reincarnation (I almost want to say something old-fashioned, like "vapours") feel centered on the pain of losing someone in war, or of losing a child, perhaps in war. When I was very little I had the tendency to speak with an English accent, which was pretty strange coming out of a kid in Ohio in the late fifties. There was a dance I always did, too, with crossing sticks that I pretended were swords. Years later I saw the same dance done by Scottish highlanders.

My memory-feeling-vapours are all over the place time-wise. One is of waiting in a forest for someone to come from the castle. There was an overwhelming memory-vision set in a small square where I was saying goodbye to a soldier I clearly loved who wore a gray cape. That dream repeated itself constantly when I was a child and as a teen-ager.

I visited England for the first time when I was nineteen, with my parents. My room looked out on the same square; it's in Kensington. London is as familiar to me as if I grew up there. I can walk through places I've never been in this lifetime and know what is just around the corner. I never had that experience in France, although I've probably spent more time in France than in Great Britain.

Regarding Sophie and France, though, there is a very strong prenatal tie-in. Most women get cravings for food when pregnant. My craving while pregnant with Sophie was for Napoleonic history. It was obsessive and felt as if it came from my belly. We lived in New York City when I was carrying her and I usually walked home from work. I had to stop at the bookstore every day to look at the history books with pictures of Josephine, and I bought all the paperbacks I could tote around and read them. It got so bad my husband flew us to Paris so we could visit Napoleon's tomb. There were no profound experiences tomb-side, nothing like wild kicking in the womb. But I did feel sated and that was a comfort.

Sophie and I have known each other from before, though. Intensely, like a mother and daughter, over and over. Rose, who is a miracle of laughter and light, does not come through quite that way. She is more my teacher in this life, if that makes any sense. Everyone who meets her thinks she's an Irish elf. She seems in some ways more advanced than Sophie, although she didn't develop verbally quite so young. Sometimes I get the odd feeling she was the person I was waiting for in the forest.

April

This morning Sophie climbed in bed with me for a morning cuddle. She asked me if I heard a jingling noise. After listening for a while I couldn't, and told her. She said that well, it was just the fairies, or angels. She wasn't sure which. She said that they were over by Rosie's crib and that you could see them best when you closed your eyes. They all carry lights and you could see the lights through your eyelids. This might just be the product of an amazing imagination, but I thought you'd like it.

I "saw" Sophie standing at the foot of our bed on our honeymoon, and had always thought it was pretty scary and not something to mention to anyone. In fact, it's worried me a lot because I thought it was a vision, perhaps, and that she wouldn't live beyond the age I saw her at. So it was a real comfort to read what you've written in *Soul Trek* regarding how children-to-be often appear as an older child, not as a baby.

I nearly had a miscarriage while pregnant with Sophie. It was close to the end of my first trimester and I started to bleed heavily. I was out of town at the time, for work, and called my doctor at home who told me it was no doubt a miscarriage. I didn't give up and found a doctor in the town I was staying in who suggested I spend the night with my legs up and hold an ice pack over my belly, which I did. I also talked with the baby the entire night, and told her we would respect whatever she chose to do but that we wanted her very much to live and be with us. My husband, who happened to be traveling with me, thought I was a little nuts, but when we went to see the doctor the next morning, there was still a heartbeat.

June

Sophie still talks with her grandpa. She told me a couple of days ago that "he is with me, you know." In fact, she says he is with her all the time. I am worried.

I guess I'm concerned on two levels. One is the ordinary level of a mother wanting her kid to fit in, with some worry that Sophie, who is extremely sensitive to what other children say, will start telling kids about what her dead grandpa is saying to her the way she does here, and that she's going to be labeled weird. We're in a new town, she's starting kindergarten in the fall, and she's an odd-duck anyway because she's so smart and seems much older than her peers. They already, with surprising frequency, tell her she talks "funny." So, you take a kid like that and have her discussing the latest report from dear, dead Grandpa, and you've got trouble.

The other side deals with the man himself. I loved my father-in-law a great deal. He was a family man to the core, put four kids through college on a factory worker's salary, instilled an eager desire to learn in all his kids...he was a great guy. But since his death there has been a sense of frustration coming from him. I felt it, Ted has felt it, and so has Richard, one of Ted's older brothers.

Sophie's Grandpa was an extremely frustrated man in life, always trying to express himself to you and stumbling all over the place as he did so. He had huge troubles with personal communication, not really due to any defect, although I guess he was dyslexic and had Attention Deficit Disorder. But it was like there was a pressure valve that was on too tight. He would tell you his opinion, and if you agreed with him he just kept on arguing. He had a dreadful childhood and it never seemed to get soothed to the point that the hurt in his heart could sit down and just be there, it had to push-push all the time. So it's hard for those who knew him to imagine him not fighting whatever situation he's in now.

This troubles me because I don't have even a glimmer of understanding as to why he is "coming through" Sophie as much as he is, unless it's a version of his continued need to be heard. But I also can't imagine him ever doing anything intentionally harmful to her. I have always believed that when we die our souls return to a more perfect state so the chance of being a troublesome spirit is unlikely.

August

Sophie has been going to a special therapist for her fears, and seems to be doing better. Her empathic abilities were overwhelming her and I felt she needed support from an outside advisor. I was lucky to find this woman. She's also helping Sophie with some of her "special talents," which are interesting. Sophie sees auras, what is going on in a person. Can feel their pulse without touching. At the ripe old age of five, she has become a healer. She rubs her hands together, holds them over a person's wound or sickened part, and does...her thing.

I dislocated a kneecap and she worked on it and it's much better. She can see red spots on a person where there are problems, feels inside for trouble, bones, her poor sister's persistent constipation. The therapist is amazed. It is so important that Sophie believe this to be a gift and not something to make her strange.

November

My mother was ill and I've been out of town for quite a while. She died, I'm an only child, and it was pretty rough. Still is. In our last years we developed a fairly deep friendship. It was complex, she was a very complex woman. I think being a friend was much easier for her than being a mother. I miss her.

I was with her when she died and felt what I can only believe was her soul passing through me. It was the most incredible feeling…beyond my imagination. It was exotic and playful and interesting, my mom in essence, without the physical pain and years of family garbage she'd carried her whole life. It gave me renewed belief.

January 2001

Rose, who turned three on Saturday, has been asking for her mommy, but says it's not me. Her "other mommy." Sophie's still psychic, even after turning six. I am blessed.

March

Rose has started in on the whole past life thing. Amazing. She told me a long story about her other daddy, how he was trying to save her and her brothers and sisters and how the bad men came and shot him and then killed her and her brothers and sisters. "I died, Mom." She looked very earnest when telling me this. She also has had some "Spanish episodes" where she speaks in Spanish. Just a word here or there, nothing major, such as asking for agua instead of water, and I'm the one always babbling in French, so the Spanish word wouldn't be familiar to her.

I had a dream about her in the Spanish civil war, but who knows. It's a war I've read several books on, but I've read books on quite a few wars, as it was part of my political science major in college. Rose looks like an Irish or Scottish waif. She has very curly strawberry blond hair, green eyes, and very fair skin. She is small, her features are small. So sensing something Spanish through that face and person is odd.

Sophie continues to get stronger as a healer. I've been taking her for lessons from a Reiki healer in town. She's good. What a wacky family!

May

Rose constantly talks about violence, about her "other mommy and daddy" being killed. Today she told me that when I was a baby "before," I died in a fire. She discusses these things so easily it's a little eerie.

Regarding Sophie and memory, most of it is fogging, although she finds comfort in talking about it and asking me what she used to say. The spirit side that has lingered is her healing skill, and that actually is becoming stronger. She very much can read my mind and I can feel it when she's doing it, almost like footprints in there. It's great fun. Rose is getting there, too. So we haven't lost everything with time and I'm grateful for that.

My mother's death in October has had a powerful effect on my girls, although none of us is "in touch" with mom. One day I was very blue, missing my mother dreadfully, and wondering where she is right now. But I didn't say anything about it to my children. Rose piped up with, "Don't be sad, Grandma's going to be a ballet dancer."

My mom would have loved that.

September

A couple of nights ago I was tucking Rose in bed and we were having some time to just be together. She said, "I love you so much, Mommy. 'Member when you kept having all those babies die? They kept sending you babies and they all kept dying? Then they said 'Let's send Rosie-girl.' And I said I love you, Mommy, most of all, and I left my other mommy and I came to be with you."

My husband and I started trying to have another baby when Sophie was about two, maybe earlier because we wanted the second to be born when Soph was two. I conceived right away, and had a miscarriage. And then another. And another. It seemed like I'd get pregnant, it would hold for three months, and then I'd lose the baby. I figured it was because I was older (forty) and yet I somehow had faith it would work out okay. Anyway, Rose knows nothing about this, nor does her sister. But it fits with what she said. And by the way, we've never called her "Rosie-girl."

November

I have a question about something that came up with Rose and wonder if you've ever heard of this (it's new to me). Last night Rose was smiling and nodding and saying something softly and I asked her what she was doing. She said, "Oh, I was talking with my baby. We were talking about you. You know, the baby I'm going to have."

Been there?

29

Closing the Circle

o o o o o o o o o o o o o o o o o o o o o o o o o o o o o o o o

Are there any accounts from the children who had some sort of pre-natal communication with their mothers, about these contacts after they're born? Do they, too, remember?

——*question from a Hungarian professor*

I have only stories to offer…not cold hard facts but soft, warm stories, quite useless for persuading anyone of the reality of souls and pre-birth communication. True research in this area is long overdue, and I hope there are people curious and patient enough to design and carry out the studies needed. However, it is not statistics but stories that make new ideas live and gradually render them familiar and understandable.

Still, one wishes for some kind of proof that pre-birth communication is real and emanates from the unborn soul. I think the best evidence we can hope to find will come in cases where a child's memory dovetails with a parent's experience of prenatal contact.

Several years ago, I was delighted to receive the question that heads this chapter. I had not found such a case, but I was confident that if unborn souls communicate, the stories would appear. Already there were published accounts of people who recalled (while in hypnosis) hovering over their pregnant mother and trying to influence her choices of food, rest, and so on. But this is only half the circle, and I had not been able to match a prenatal memory with a parent's experience.

Since then, I've gathered a few stories that come closer—tantalizingly close—to completing the circuit. Emily's observation of her little girl talking to "the baby she's going to have" reminded me of this intriguing account from a Midwestern mother of three:

Beverly*: The green rocking chair

I remember talking to someone at night when I was six years old. The little girl was sitting in my rocking chair. I remember her telling me that I would be her Mommy, and she told me things she would do when she got here. My mother remembers that time too. She often said she would come up the stairs thinking I was talking to my sister, and planning to tell us we should be sleeping. She'd find me sitting up in bed talking—and my sister sound asleep. She said it made the hair stand straight up on the back of her neck.

I now have a fourteen-year-old daughter, Cassie, as well as two younger sons. When she was three and a half, Cassie asked me if I remembered when she used to come and see me at night. She asked where her green rocking chair was! I still have the chair and my daughter remembered it in detail. It had one broken rod in the back, which my grandfather fixed when I was around nine. Cassie asked why the chair was different. This really shook me up. Now she doesn't remember ever asking me that question.

Three-and-a-half seems to be the golden age for children's revelations. Beverly says her daughter no longer has any memory of the night-time visits, but may still "remember remembering" the rocking chair. In the next story, the hint of a link back to pre-birth communication is slim, but suggestive.

Judith: "I wanted to come before"

When I was nineteen, I became pregnant. I was married and loved my husband very much, but we were poor, I was in college, and we had barely enough to get by. More than anything, I wanted to finish college and go on to graduate school. I cried when I found out I was pregnant, and wanted this child to go away, because I was not ready.

I miscarried, and would never have had an abortion because I am a devout Catholic Latina. After the miscarriage, I became deathly ill and required surgery to remove a ruptured ovarian cyst and stop internal hemorrhaging. But I kept dreaming of this beautiful, curly-haired little boy. I knew he was a soul in heaven who wanted to be born. I knew he was mine.

He kept appearing to me over the years, silently and patiently walking toward me. I kept rejecting and suppressing the dream, because I truly believed I would not be a good mother, and wanted to dedicate myself to my career. My own mother had often told me that I would not be a good mother.

Eventually, after finishing my Ph.D. and getting a faculty position at a major university, I met my new husband under very stressful and painful circumstances. I wasn't even sure of our relationship, but I was in the career of my choice, and I knew I could raise a child. I let my guard down and Paul was conceived when I was thirty-four. When he was born, I fell instantly in love with him and was willing to do anything for him, even be a single mom. I actually began to hate my husband, and falling in love with him again required a lot of healing.

Little Paul became the focus of my healing, because my love for him sustained me in all circumstances. He grew to have curly black hair, which now he keeps cropped and straight. He's the love of my life. In the process, I got a "bonus baby," his little sister, a beautiful child who came as a total surprise soon after Paul.

I am sure my son Paul is the little boy in the dream. In fact, when he was about five years old, he said something very strange: "Mommy, I wanted to come before, but you didn't want me then." When he said that, I almost fell down with surprise.

Dr. Gladys Taylor McGarey's book *The Physician Within You* includes a compelling account of soul connections. The story of Susan links a child's memory back to a loving bond made before birth. Susan found herself pregnant at seventeen, just as she was about to enter college. She decided to talk to the child, whom she perceived as a girl. Speaking softly, she explained why it was the wrong time for her to have a baby, promising, "You will only be away a little while. We will be together again." In her third month, she miscarried.

Two years later, Susan's best friend Fran, who was older and happily married, had her first baby. The night of the birth, Susan woke to hear a child's voice announcing, "Mama, I'm coming back."

"As I heard the child's voice I jumped out of bed," says Susan. "I could almost feel her presence...A thrill of joy swept over me. In that moment I knew it was my little girl—a promise fulfilled. I could hardly wait to see her. Nobody thought anything of my rushing over to the hospital. I was 'family.'

"From the beginning we had this special bond," Susan says, "like we both knew of our previous connection. I thought of her as my child. She would throw up her arms to greet me with the happiest smile. When she was able to toddle she would rush into my arms."

Wishful thinking? When the little girl was three, her mother was again pregnant and Susan was visiting. Sitting on Susan's lap, the child suddenly asked, "Do you remember when I was in your tummy?"

"No, honey," Susan replied, "you were in your mother's tummy."

The child shook her head. "Not that first time."

Uncertain of how to respond, Susan asked, "What did you do in my tummy?"

Sadly the little girl replied, "I cried."

"Why did you cry?"

"Because they said I couldn't stay. They said it wasn't the time. They pulled me back."

"Who were they?" Susan finally asked.

"The same ones that brought me to you."

Among all the stories related to me, the following one is perhaps the most compelling as evidence for the reality of pre-existence.

Wendy: "No, Mom...I was in Spirit"

My youngest son, Philip, described events which occurred before he was born, before he was even conceived—facts which he had no way of knowing other than by somehow being there. Philip was about three at the time and talking well. I pulled out my flute to show my boys. I hadn't played it for about six years because of moving around the world and storing things away. The flute had come out of storage, so I played a few tunes. Then Philip stated, "Gee, Mom, I remember when you used to play that all the time."

I stopped and looked at him and remarked, "Phil, that's not possible because I haven't played the flute since way before you were born!"

His comment was, "I remember you used to always play it in that house where you stepped down into the wood-stove room." He then described a room which indeed was accurate, three houses prior to our present house in which he was born.

I replied, "I know which room you're talking about, and that's the living room of where I used to live in Pennsylvania, but you were not born yet when I was in that house and you never visited that house either."

That's when he nearly shocked me right out of my skin. My three-year-old blurted out, "No, Mom, I wasn't alive yet, I was in Spirit." Plain and simple to understand—but "in Spirit" was not a term I had used with him at that point. It caused me to ponder the truth of his words and I had no argument left, since he was able to describe in detail an event of my life before he was born.

Phil said a lot of things that day and onward. He claims to have picked me as his mother. That was another of his funny comments—because I had waited ten years before I had children in my first marriage, and I thought I was the one who chose to have him. He's a wonder to me on a spiritual level and a catalyst to my studies. I began an intense study of the Bible and all spiritual writings as a result of some of his comments. I always feared I'd teach him wrong things, so I studied Spirit matters in order not to mislead him due to my own lack of understanding.

He remembered details which I later had to validate with my mother, to check on his funny words of pre-birth memories. For example, the names of a horse and a pig that my mother had as pets in her childhood, which was spent on the same street where Phil remembers me playing the flute. Since I lived in Germany and then Maryland, my parents had little access to these grandchildren, so I ruled out the possibility of Grandmom telling him, and later confirmed that she never talked to him of those things.

Before I had children, I would come home from work and play my flute in the room Phil described. One night I had a very strange sensation, and I began playing better than I was capable of doing. It went on for a minute or two and I threw the flute down on the couch because it felt like I was not playing it—someone else was. It was a spooky feeling yet I wasn't really too afraid, because I knew who it could be.

That particular house happened to be right up the street from my great great grandfather's farm, and he was said to have been a flute player. I always wondered if that night, my great great grandfather came to visit me, because I was so close to his homestead, and it felt like something came into me and took over the flute and my fingers were going faster than ever before or since.

Phil seems old for his young age. He blurts out statements that are so profound, that cause the adults in the room to stop short and think. Yet he's not so good in the academic school type activities. I keep waiting for his potential and wisdom to be reflected somewhat on his report card. Teachers have repeated the comment, they were surprised he passed the test because they were sure he wasn't paying attention! He is a dreamer and daydreams a lot.

My final analysis, after Phil's comments and much reading on such subjects, is that I suppose it is possible that it was my son who was there, that strange evening (it still gives me goosebumps thinking about it), and possibly my son is some ancestor's spirit who was reincarnated.

I can never know, but my mind is open to that possibility.

30

The Homesick Soul

o o o o o o o o o o o o o o o o o o o o o o o o o o o o o o o o o o

In view of the memory which works perfectly well during an out-of-body or near-death experience, which survives the physical demise of both body and brain (as in confirmed past life recall), and the continuity of understanding and even wisdom demonstrated by new beings at any stage from before conception to after birth, it seems obvious to me that memory is immaterial yet continuing, and must be an aspect of soul.

—David Chamberlain, Ph.D. (Personal communication)

There are people who live with homesickness for a place before birth. They remember an existence where harmony was real and peace was possible. Some of them remember trying to resist being pulled or pushed out of that place and into this life.

In this final chapter we'll meet people who approached the world reluctantly. Their stories help us understand why arriving souls need much gentleness and reassurance in adjusting to the conditions of earth life. They also give us some perspective on why souls might decide to turn back instead of completing the journey to birth.

In her autobiography, *Second Sight*, medical intuitive Judith Orloff describes her distress at finding herself trapped in the womb and cut off from "home." Her story shows that even before birth a child may be suffering from homesickness. It suggests, too, that the remembered home is personal, perhaps unique to each individual.

When Judith's mother was five months pregnant, the baby's life was threatened by large fibroid tumors growing on the outside of the womb. There was no choice but to go ahead with surgery to remove them. In hypnosis many years later, Judith recalled what she experienced during the operation. The terrible intensity of sounds and sensations caused her to "awaken prematurely" in the womb. She found herself in "a dark, claustrophobic space, with warm, salty fluid swishing past a strange form that felt like it was me—yet I didn't recognize myself." In a panic, she struggled to leave and return home, though she could not picture what was "home."

Unable to break free of the alien environment, she escaped into a dream, where she found herself in front of a farmhouse, being greeted by a woman with long blond braids who seemed strikingly familiar. Judith recalled her relief at seeing this woman, as well as her husband and two teenage sons. These people felt like her real family, and the farmhouse surrounded by green hills felt like home. In the dream, they talked and laughed together, easing the tension of her predicament.

Judith continued to visit this comforting family in prenatal dreams, although she was never able to identify who they were or why they were so familiar. She longed to remain with them, but they encouraged her to stay where she was: "Reassuring me that I would be all right and that they loved me, these dear people…talked me through the remainder of my often disturbing stay in the womb." Judith's remembered experience raises an intriguing possibility. Perhaps some of the dream-children and vision-children who never show up in this reality are members of other families that we love and belong to, elsewhere.

Helen Wambach was a psychologist who experimented with hypnotizing groups of people and regressing them to pre-birth. Analyzing the reports of their experiences, she found that sixty-eight percent of her subjects recalled feeling "reluctant, anxious or resigned" at the prospect of leaving the pre-conception state and coming to birth.[1] There is a primordial trauma that predates the birth trauma. Children who carry these memories may feel they don't belong here; they may be burdened with nostalgia and long to return home. Their loneliness is increased when they try to describe what they remember and meet only baffled incomprehension. Some are even punished for expressing ideas that run counter to their family's beliefs. I hope that sharing these stories will help such children to be heard and comforted.

Even those who come willingly may suffer from homesickness for the pre-existence. I can never forget my three-year-old son saying to me, "Let's go home." When I asked him where home was, he pointed upward and replied, "Far, far away. Up in the sky. This the dirt place. Our home up there."

Greta* has no conscious memories of such a home, but throughout her childhood she treasured what she calls the "going home dream." She explains: "When I was a tiny child, I had the dream every night. I would go home with the light; that's all I can call it. It was like going home with a parent. The light was pure white, silvery white. At about age twelve I had my last going home dream, and the light was telling me goodbye. I cannot say why I needed these dreams, but my childhood was not the best. I know that when I die, the light will take me home."

It is uncomfortable to face evidence that our children might not be thrilled with the prospect of being in this world. Can we ever bring the experience of earth life into line with the soul's desires? These stories deepen my awareness of the need for much more tenderness and communication with our children, from pre-conception right through childhood.

Beyond feeling "reluctant, anxious, or resigned" at the prospect of earth life, there are people who remember fighting hard to refuse the experience. For the next two recallers, their soul memories have had an enormous effect upon them, and both express an intense wish to return to that other existence.

Mike Perkins: Every day I long for a time that has gone by

I have pre-birth memories. I didn't want to come back, but was forced. I was told I would not remember anything. However, I am a very stubborn person and refused to be dumb—I remember quite a bit. I remember being commanded, "Wake up, wake up!" I didn't want to wake up; I was comfortable. I was told I had to go back. I didn't want to, I begged and pleaded, but was told I had no choice. I was very angry because of this. I was assured that things are different now, but I still didn't want to go.

The person I was talking to had golden curly hair and fair skin, and glowed. I don't remember anyone else there. Everything else was dark like space without stars.

The next thing I know, I am suffocating, fighting to find a way out. I remember being born, and then I was in an elevator, lying on my stomach looking to the left corner of the elevator, and there was the person. I told him that I have to remember. I was afraid that if I didn't, I would do the wrong thing and would not be able to return. I asked, "How will I know to do good?" He said, "Don't worry. You'll be fine, you won't remember any of this." I asked if I would see him again if I needed help. He said, "No, not until you return, you'll live a long life." Then he was gone.

I kept thinking about this through the next year so I wouldn't forget. I remember not being able to understand anyone and getting aggravated because I didn't think I would ever learn how to speak this language. I remember sitting in a walker outdoors, maybe a year old, and I wanted so badly to keep all my memories so that when I got to be thirty years old I could find something or do something. Then I thought of how long it would take to get to thirty, and gave up trying to remember all of my pre-birth.

I didn't like the idea of growing up again and going through listening to adults, being told what to do and when to do it. However, I stopped trying to remember and started to just exist. I forgot all but what I've related here, and can't remember what I wanted to find or look for. I have spent my life searching for something that I don't know what it is. At age thirty-seven, I still do not want to be here, never have and never will. Every day I long for a time that has gone by…

Soul memory is a two-edged sword, both a blessing and a burden. Perhaps we need to forget, so we can adapt to the conditions of this world. Most of the people who have memories of pre-existence speak of their homesickness for that place, but also realize that they are fortunate to have first-hand knowledge of the soul's reality. Remembering other realms, they are not afraid of death. But still, to remember an existence that felt like the soul's true home means living in this world as a displaced person. These feelings are very much like the dissonance—the "not fitting in any more"—that afflicts many survivors of a near-death experience. The next story makes this crushingly clear.

Dawn D. Lafady: I miss it with all my heart

I really thought I was the only one in the world who could remember. I am very excited to hear about the others. Are their memories a lot like mine? I have waited a lifetime to discover another like myself.

I clearly remember like it was this morning. There was more light and love and happiness than you could ever imagine, it's more than our universe could hold. The only way that I could describe it is if you were to take all the love you have ever felt in your entire life, and combine it all together, it would measure as one little grain of sand compared to all the sand found on all the beaches and deserts of the world.

I remember being within a golden city full of the brightest white light, and the light was love and I also was a part of that light, like a large ocean of light and love with countless others. Then I was pulled away and became separate, as if you took a dropper and pulled out of the ocean one single drop. I am still the ocean, but yet now a separate single drop.

I was carried away by a compassionate, almost father-like figure. I will be so bold and say Jesus Christ, and he was also light and there is no physical form. I was held and carried away as if flying at great speed until we were into the heavenly stars, just as you see when you look up. I was then placed on top of a very small planet-like place. All that was there was a rocky dirt path that started from the top and spiraled all the way around this planet to the bottom.

I became of physical form the moment I was placed there atop this path. I cried to him as if he were my father, "No! Please, I don't want to leave," like a child when a parent drops a small child off somewhere and they desperately don't want their parent to leave. I was in a long white robe with a golden rope of some sort tied loosely around my waist. I also had a very large staff taller than myself. I was crushed and broken-hearted and pleaded that I didn't want to go.

The light being Jesus was very bright and hovered way above me like a bright star. I remember my tears and sadness. He said to me telepathically in a male voice, "You must go, my child." He said it with all the love and compassion in the universe. My love for him and for the home I was leaving was just as intense.

I became frightened and at that moment I became angry and then in a tantrum rage I picked up my staff and with both my hands I raised it above my head and I screamed No! striking my staff as hard as I could against a large boulder that lay to the left of this path. The very instant I struck the rock, it melted and turned into water and at that instant I became a part of that water and very quickly flowed down this spiral path to the bottom like a raging river, and it was then I was born. I was born an angry child.

I have never forgotten nor will I ever forget. It's been a part of me since the beginning of time. From the moment I could express myself and form sentences I cried to my family that I wanted to go back to the love. They didn't understand until I was old enough to explain what I meant.

Throughout my life, whenever I reflect on it I see myself as I am now; as a child I saw myself as a child and so on. When I try to understand more about what happened to me, I can't; but some-times I wonder if I was crying not only about having to leave my loving home, but perhaps I knew where I was going because I had been here before, and that created a greater fear and sadness on coming back.

I don't know why I was allowed to remember. I know I was *allowed* and it was not just some freak thing that happened. I have made mistakes in my life just like others, maybe more. I have had many tragedies in my life just like others. I can tell you that knowing leaves a comparison between there and here, and life here is very painful. I have had many joys and blessings in my life, but life in comparison seems like detention and I am just waiting until I've been called to go home. I miss it with all my heart.

Kathy lives in the Midwest and owns her own business; she is married and the mother of twin teenage girls. As a child with pre-birth memories, she gradually realized that her different viewpoint set her apart from family and playmates and caused deep loneliness. There is so much to contemplate in her description of a primordial state of pure being. It seems the perfect place to end this step of our exploration.

Kathy: I Was a Part of Everything

I remember coming here in spirit form, coming together into the body form and reluctantly floating down to this planet. This powerful experience from before my birth has affected everything I am today. It has given me insights, and peace that is hard to explain, yet also causes me grief when I see what horrors mankind is capable of.

I remember as a small child being very confused when I watched people. I assumed they all had the same memory I had, that they understood we were all part of the one and connected to one another and how we all affect one another. I couldn't understand how even my little playmates could do cruel things to their friends or their brothers or sisters, if they remembered what I did.

My memory has never left me, nor has it ever changed in any way. The only thing that changes is that as I grow and my vocabulary increases, I am better able to describe it even though I still have a long way to go and doubt it ever can be done in the confines of the English language. It is as ingrained in me as my own fingerprints. In fact, that experience and memory is much more real and vivid to me even now, than my actual reality around me as a human being. I have never doubted it, although I must admit there have been frustrating periods in my life when I felt the world was nothing but a loony bin, when I have wondered if someone actually gave me this memory as a joke just to see how I handled it. Nonetheless, it is more real to me than anything else is and it has shaped who I am today.

When I was four, my father asked me what was the first thing I remembered. I told him simply, in four-year-old language, that I remembered coming here and getting a body and then coming to the planet. I vaguely recall the look on his face, which I didn't understand at the time. To me, there was nothing odd about my memory and I figured everyone would remember coming here.

I was about seven when I realized I was the odd man out. I became very private about my memory and considered it a gift from God. I thought how wonderful it was that I remember what it is like before birth. I know for a fact that there is life before and after and in between. I remember it flawlessly. I have no fear of dying, and that allows me to live more freely. So many people are afraid to live because of their fears of death.

Having a pre-birth memory did cause some trouble for me. From the very beginning, I longed for my "other" who I knew was not with me. I also constantly searched for a "big brother," so insistently that I accused my parents of having a son before me (I'm the eldest), and doing away with him. For some reason, "big brother" was who I needed to find first. (There is a story that goes with this, including a dream of meeting a man whom I had never seen before and then later met, who confirmed he was very much my big brother and teacher and who also led me to the one whom I now know as my "other.")

Other problems the memory caused in my young age included arguing with my grandparents about their Bible belt religion, and knowing that the Bible only contained half-truths and they were taking it too literally. I was eight or nine years old at the time and nearly got my mouth washed out with soap.

I would look at my parents and wonder who they really were and how I came to be with them, and long for a home that wasn't where I was living. In my frustration I would sometimes stamp my feet on the ground and yell up at the sky, "Why can't you come with me?" or, "Tell me why I came here again!"

Mostly, I found I was incredibly lonely. Even though I felt connected to all, in this reality I was the different one and it seems I spent my entire childhood trying to fit in and just be part of the crowd. But I had a hard time making sense of what some of my teen-aged friends would do for a good time, so that often, even when I was with them I still wasn't "with them."

One Cell in the Body of God

In the beginning, I remember simply being in space. There was another who accompanied me, but I had been left on my own in order to prepare. Explaining "what" I was at that point is difficult for I have yet to find words that would accurately describe an experience not understood in this reality.

I was a part of everything and everything was a part of me. I was aware of the connection that flowed through me to all life and all forms of life. Although I was a part of the "all," I was still "me." The center of my being, the perspective from which I viewed and experienced things, was as it is in this reality—as though I still had my heart and my mind, or rather my soul, even though I was not in a body form. I was still uniquely me.

I remember looking all around me and being able to see all around me at the same time. As I peered into the darkness, I became aware of the enormity and the simplicity of it all. It was like looking into nothing and everything at once.

I was aware and could feel that I was completely connected to everything in the universe, as though I was one individual cell in the body of God, with each cell serving a different purpose, small and minute, yet still individually important in our own right. I realized that all the living things in the universe, be they animal, human, or yet undiscovered, were connected in a unique dance, whether the life-form is aware of it or not.

I remember looking into the vastness of space and realizing the incredible magnitude of mysteries and knowledge and complexities, but also that it was as simple or as complicated as I chose to make it.

I realized that in this state of being I could access a "universal library," and through this connectedness, I could learn anything I cared to know. I could also feel that which was around me. For example if there was extreme joy, I was aware of it; destruction or sadness, I was aware of that too. All I had to do was put my attention towards something and all the information learned by the "whole" would be given to me.

I saw that I could learn everything there was to know about something as experienced so far by the whole, but first, I had to evolve enough to know what to ask. I was aware that the knowledge was beyond the imagination, but also that it was my responsibility to experience and contribute to the whole. Answers to so many of life's burning questions were all within my reach, but I had to grow and learn how and what to ask for, and in my growing, I contributed to the "whole" as well. The "whole" was also continually evolving and growing.

In this state I was without any fear. There was a calm I have never experienced since and a quiet that doesn't exist on this planet. I don't remember ego. Things simply *were*. We were all equal, no need for ego. Then, I began to come together.

I remember the feeling well. It was as if millions of tiny pieces of any tangible part of the universe came rushing towards my center being. A feeling similar to when one's leg goes numb and the blood is beginning to circulate again, except there was no pain. Like a million tiny bubbles coming together from the far reaches of space until they all converged upon me and created one body around me.

I remember floating there in space, pressing my arms against my thighs and reassuring myself that "this is just another form of being. It's okay. It's just different." I remember I didn't like the fact that I couldn't see all around me any more. I felt very limited in this form, although my heart and mind and soul were still connected to everything else.

As I floated there, I looked directly above me into what as a child I would call a "silver cloud." I was aware that the other being who came with me was on the other side of that "cloud," but I was not to go back. I turned my head to the left and looked down below my shoulder. Below me was the most beautiful, vivid blue planet, breathtaking against the inky blackness of space.

But even among all of this beauty I became aware of another fact: I really didn't want to go to this planet. This was when I felt my first strong emotion, and it was one of nearly dread. The problem was that no matter how I felt, I knew I had "volunteered." I had a choice whether or not to come; however, I also remember that I felt like I really didn't have a choice. I had to come for some very important purpose or need. So, after a short time of contemplation and becoming familiar in this body form, I slowly began to float down towards this planet, watching it grow closer and closer as I glided downwards.

I do not remember anything about being in the womb or being born. As I floated down to this planet, it was as if everything resolved into blackness.

Sharing the Secret

For the last eleven years I have co-owned a medical boutique that caters primarily to breast cancer ladies. Although I love my job immensely, I am still unsure that this is what I am supposed to do. In relaxing and actually sharing my pre-birth memory with a select few who seemed sincere and honest enough to listen, I have found myself slowly becoming more at home with me and this body. I think it's all just part of the process. Having my experience published where someone else like me might happen to read it and realize they are not the only one, makes me feel like I'm beginning to hit on a part of why I came here in the first place. I can't tell you the comfort I have received in finding another like me and who I know understands.

It's really too beautiful a secret to keep all to ourselves.

About the Author

Elisabeth Hallett is an independent researcher who believes people's experiences are filled with clues to the mysteries of life and death. With a background in Psychology and nursing (plus a mini-career as a yoga teacher), she turned to writing and research after the birth of her first child. *In The Newborn Year* (published 1992) highlights the full rainbow of postpartum changes in awareness. *Soul Trek* (1995) is an in-depth study of Pre-Birth Communication; and the present work continues Elisabeth's exploration of this exciting field. Never knowing where the trail of clues will lead her next, Elisabeth welcomes correspondence from her readers and invites them to visit her website at **www.light-hearts.com**. She lives with her husband Nicholas and daughter Roselyn in the Bitterroot Valley of Montana. Her son, Devin, is a university student.

ENDNOTES

Chapter One: The Shiver Sign

1. See especially *Coming From The Light: Spiritual Accounts of Life Before Life* by Sarah Hinze (Pocket Books, 1997) and *Cosmic Cradle: Souls Waiting in the Wings for Birth*, by Elizabeth Carman and Neil Carman, Ph.D. (Sunstar, 2000). It's intriguing that Sarah Hinze and I were researching pre-birth communication at the same time, unknown to one another. When the time is ripe for an idea, it tends to emerge in several places at once.

Chapter Two: Soul Memory

1. Michael Maguire maintains an expanding list of people who have pre-birth memories and are interested in connecting with others. Contact him at: 25 Kirkston Place, Pine Mountain, Queensland, Australia, 4306 or Phone (07) 3201-5834

2. Some of the stories in this chapter first appeared on Sarah Hinze's message board. Special thanks to Sarah for allowing me to connect with contributors to her website, **www.prebirth.com**

Chapter Three: Pre-Conception Visits

1. David Brunner shares other visionary stories on his website, Stepping Stones, at **http://steppingstones.to**

Chapter Four: Windows on Pre-Existence

1. Portions of the poem by Silvan Waffle are reproduced with the kind permission of the author. The full poem follows:

Made in secret

They line up
little people yet to be.
Unborn faces in a crowd of futures.
None of them exist apart from a miracle
and yet how does that make them
so different from me?
They are all in halves right now.
A few dozen in her, determined.
Many millions inside of me
still fracturing in multitudes of possibilities
each one ready to collide with certainty
deciding a body
and framework of a personality.
The combinations could give forth one more
or maybe three
into full life and birth.
Yet now I can't help picturing them
all in a line waiting
in some shadowy star-shined
vestibule in space
pacing quietly, slowly
maybe hoping
praying
that we will seek them.
Already we have reached out
arms blind
taking and holding three
one that went in silence and mystery
two who have flourished like green shoots
as different as rose and sunflower
both lovely beneath the summer heat.
How daunting the task

of shedding all my sunlight for their nurture!
Can my garden
hold even these two blooms?
Yet how enticing the thought
of calling another bursting seed
across the boundary
of blood and flesh.

Copyright Silvan Waffle 1995

Chapter Five: Conception: Energy Encounters

1. The father's story is from *The Mother-to-be's Dream Book: Understanding the Dreams of Pregnancy*, by Raïna Paris (Warner Books, 2000).

2. Reverend Linda Bedre maintains a practice in Houston, assisting people to heal who have pre-conception, womb, birth, and early life memories. She can be contacted at anewway@earthlink.net

Chapter Seven: Communing in Pregnancy

1. Robert Van de Castle's comment appeared in his article published in December, 2000, on the internet site Dream Time. Dr. Van de Castle shared my fascination with a news item in TIME Magazine, June 26, 2000. It described a study carried out at Johns Hopkins university in which 104 pregnant women were interviewed and asked to foretell their babies' sex before any prenatal testing was carried out. They were asked whether their guess was based on folklore, the way they were carrying the baby, a dream or just a feeling. The results? "Of the women who based their forecast on a feeling or dream, 71% were correct, and all the women who cited a dream were right."

It would be instructive to run a similar study on fathers, for they too can be intuitive, without the direct physical contact with their child. As Michael Maguire says, "I just knew I was going to have a daughter. It was as if this was being communicated to me somehow throughout the pregnancy."

2. Cassandra Eason: I highly recommend her books for more stories of the telepathic bond between parent and child. *A Mother's Instincts* (Aquarian/Thorsons, 1992) and *Mother Love* (Robinson Publishing, 1998) are particularly good. The latter is available in the United States as *The Mother Link*.

Chapter Eight: Outside Connections

1. Robert Moss describes the concept of "soul helpers" in *Dreaming True: How to Dream Your Future and Change Your Life for the Better* (Pocket Books, 2000).

Chapter Nine: Working It Out With Ezra

1. Holland Franklin, whose online presence is at **transformationdynamics.com** offers a story that independently parallels John Dye's theory about breech presentations:

I was seven and a half months pregnant with my second child and the baby was persistently in breech position. I was working with two wonderful midwives, and I also sought out the help of a woman Acupuncturist, who had been a midwife in China. She promptly told me that babies don't turn at that late point in pregnancy. My midwives said otherwise and I chose to believe them instead. I spent a week doing periodic pelvic tilt exercises, to no avail. And it didn't make any sense to me that a few minutes of inversion here and there would be enough to turn the baby around. I wondered what to do.

One afternoon, while pondering this, I was walking through my living room, when it hit me! I already had a little boy, and I had wanted a girl. In fact, this baby "felt" like a girl, and I had been kind of emotionally assuming that it was a girl. What hit me was that, perhaps, this was another little boy and he was afraid to come out because he might not be loved as a boy. I immediately looked down at my belly and spoke to the baby and said, "If you are a little boy, I want you to know that I will love you completely. It will never matter to me in the slightest that you are not a girl. I will always be there for you, and always accept you as you are." I meant it.

That was in the afternoon. The next morning when I woke up, the shape of my belly was different. When I had my next appointment with one of the midwives, she told me the baby had turned. He, Kim, had a completely normal birth at home.

Chapter Ten: The Dialogue Of Agreement

1. The lama's quote is from *The Tibetan Art of Parenting: From Before Conception Through Early Childhood,* by Anne Hubbell Maiden and Edie Farwell (Wisdom Publications, 1997).

Chapter Fourteen: Courting the Soul

1. Teresa Robertson, RN, CNM, MSN, can be reached at (303)258-3904, 3011 N Broadway Suite 32, Boulder CO 80302. Her website is at **www.birthintuitive.com**

2. Kari Henley is a writer, a producer of conferences and a personal coach for women's transformation. She can be contacted at 203-453-4716, **KariHenley@aol.com**, or 38 Munger Road, Guilford, CT 06437

Chapter Fifteen: Carry On

1. Laura Shanley is a freelance writer, poet, and author of the book *Unassisted Childbirth* (Bergin & Garvey, 1994). Her website, Bornfree! The Unassisted Childbirth Page, is found at **http://ucbirth.com**

Chapter Sixteen: The Dialogue of Acceptance

1. Dr. Joanne Klink, Ph.D., is a theologian and the author of a remarkable book, *Früher, als ich gross war*, ("Before, when I was big"), unfortunately not available in English. She presents the spontaneous memories of children recalling previous lives and existence between lives. Her books are available in Dutch and German.

2. Eve Marnie's approach to communicating with the unborn child is detailed in her book *Lovestart: Pre-Birth Bonding* (Hay House, 1992).

Chapter Seventeen: Soul and Body

1. *Ich Kann Sprechen*, by Manuel David Coudris (Goldmann Verlag, 1985) was published in English by Gateway Books, 1992 as *Diary of An Unborn Child*.

2. The Dutch maternity nurse is quoted in Joanne Klink's *Fruher, als ich gross war*.

3. The story of Nadja is found in *The Holotropic Mind: The Three Levels of Human Consciousness and How They Shape Our Lives*, by Stanislav Grof (HarperCollins, 1992).

Chapter Eighteen: Abortion

1. The story of Joel is found in *Return From Heaven: Beloved Relatives Reincarnated Within Your Family*, by Carol Bowman (HarperCollins, 2001).

2. The story of the woman haunted by traumatic womb memories is related by David Chamberlain, Ph.D. in the Journal of Prenatal and Perinatal Psychology and Health Volume 14, Number 1-2, Fall/Winter 1999.

3. The young woman's story is found in Chapter Five of *The Physician Within You*, copyright 1997 by Gladys Taylor McGarey. This chapter

is a wonderful resource on the use of communication in unwelcome pregnancies.

Chapter Nineteen: Jilly's Story

1. The Post Abortion Stress Syndrome Support Site, provides support and comfort to all women after an abortion, and can be found online at **http://www.afterabortion.com**

Chapter Twenty: No Guarantees

1. The experiment with pregnant women is cited by David Chamberlain, Ph.D., in *The Mind of Your Newborn Baby* (North Atlantic Books, 1998).

Chapter Twenty-One: Dakota's Story

1. Kara writes: Our online presence can be seen at **www.kotapress.com**. On our site, we hope you find helpful information, good poetry, and some inspiration to get through the hard times.

Chapter Twenty-Five: Listen to the Children

1. The account of Nick's memories is found in *His Bright Light: The Story of Nick Traina*, by Danielle Steel (Random House/The Nick Traina Foundation, 1998).

2. Jacqueline du Pre's prescient remark is recorded in *A Genius in the Family*, by Hilary du Pre and Piers du Pre (Chatto & Windus, 1997). American editions of this marvelous biography are titled *Hilary and Jackie*.

3. Lesta Bertoia later included this beautiful story, with many additional details, in her book, *Somewhere Between Kindergarten and God: Mini-Memoirs About the Mundane and the Mystical* (Hampton Roads Publishing Company, 2001). As the subtitle suggests, Lesta's book is a

revelation of what it's like to balance everyday life with the awareness of being an immortal soul.

Chapter Thirty: The Homesick Soul

1. The thought-provoking statistic is found in Helen Wambach's *Life Before Life* (Bantam Books, 1979).

References

ACKNOWLEDGMENTS OF COPYRIGHTED MATERIAL

The author gratefully acknowledges permission to reprint excerpts from the following publications:

Epigraph: From *The Last Days of Socrates* by Plato, translated by Hugh Tredennick (Penguin Classics, Second revised edition 1969) © Hugh Tredennick. Reprinted by permission of the publisher.

From *The Near-Birth Experience: A Journey to the Center of Self,* © 2000 by Jerry Bongard. Appears by permission of the publisher, Marlowe & Company.

From *The Tibetan Art of Parenting: From Before Conception Through Early Childhood,* © Anne Hubbell Maiden and Edie Farwell, 1997. Reprinted with permission of Wisdom Publications, 199 Elm St., Somerville MA 02144 U.S.A., **www.wisdompubs.org**

From *Parenting Begins Before Conception* by Carista Luminare-Rosen, Ph.D., Healing Arts Press, Rochester, VT 05767 © 2000 by Carista Luminare-Rosen, Ph.D.

From *The Castaways: Safely in His Arms,* © 2000 by Sarah Hinze and Brent Hinze. Reprinted by permission of the authors.

From *Welcoming Spirit Home,* © 1999 by Sobonfu Somé. Reprinted with permission of New World Library. **www. newworldlibrary.com**

Dr. Jenny Wade's quotes in Chapter 17: From an article published in the Journal of Prenatal and Perinatal Psychology and Health, Volume 13, Number 2, Winter 1998 pp 142, 143: "Two Voices From the Womb: Evidence for Physically Transcendent and a Cellular Source of Fetal Consciousness" by Jenny Wade, Ph.D. By permission of the author and the editor.

Dr. David Chamberlain's quotes in Chapter 17: From an article published in the Journal of Prenatal and Perinatal Psychology and Health, Volume 14, Number 1-2, Fall/winter 1999, pp. 86-7: "Transpersonal Adventures in Prenatal and Perinatal Hypnotherapy" by David B. Chamberlain, Ph.D. By permission of the author and the editor.

Information about Dr. Myriam Szejer in Chapter 17: From APPPAH Newsletter, Summer 2001; reprinted by permission of Barbara Findeisen, author, and Maureen Wolfe, Editor.

Quote from Dr. Helen Wambach in Chapter 17: From *Life Before Life*, © 1979 by Helen Wambach. Reprinted with permission by Estate of Dr. Helen Wambach.

From *Fingers Pointing to the Moon*, © 1999 by Jane English. By permission of the author.

The California mother's story shared by Theresa Danna in Chapter 18: From an article published in EHE News, Volume 6, Number 1, March 1999, page 3: "A Comparison/Contrast Analysis of Pre-birth Experiences" by Theresa Danna. Reprinted by permission of Rhea White, Editor, and Theresa Danna.

The anecdote about Alan Watts in Chapter 24: Excerpt from *Zen Effects: The Life of Alan Watts* © 2001 by Monica Furlong, First SkyLight Paths Publishing Edition (Woodstock, VT: SkyLight Paths Publishing), $16.95+$3.75 s/h. Order by mail or call 800-

962-4544 or on-line at **www.skylightpaths.com**. Permission granted by SkyLight Paths Publishing, P.O. Box 237, Woodstock, VT 05091.

From *The Physician Within You: Medicine for the Millennium,* © 1997 by Gladys Taylor McGarey. Reprinted by kind permission of the author.

0-595-22361-3